CYTOLOGY OF THE LUNG

Foreword

Some of the first major publications on lung cytology were written by clinicians, i.e. H.H.Wandall (1944) and S. Farber et al. (1950). Now a group of experienced chest clinicians, Dr. Harubumi Kato, has published another important contribution to this difficult subject.

The clinical application of cytopathology is regarded as one of the significant advances of this century in the management of malignant tumors. Respiratory cytopathology is a compulsory part of the diagnostic work-up in any clinic dealing with cancer patients. It is hard to think of a lung clinic today without access to a respiratory cytology service.

A main advantage of this book is the concentration on the practical diagnostic approach for chest clinicians dealing with patients with respiratory symptoms. This important book deals with benign diseases and early asymptomatic cancer and discusses theoretical aspects of these subjects and methods to study the bronchil epithelium during early carcinogenesis. This volume also includes an extensive chapter on preparation techniques, various sampling methods and their relative advances in various clinical situations. Special attention has been paid to endoscopic techniques.

There is a well planned chapter on the cytomorphology of various lung tumors and important remarks on the special features of brush samples which sometimes differ considerably from those of sputum specimens. Several less common tumor types are also discussed. In addition there are several extremely useful tables summarizing the cytologic features of various alterations which present problems in differential diagnosis.

The section on the various aspects of the pathogenesis of bronchogenic cancer and corresponding epithelial cell changes is of great interest. This is also of practical importance as some precursors, particularly squamous metaplasia (dysplasia), may present difficult differential diagnostic problems. It is furthermore of great interest that the cytochemical background is described from a methodological points of view.

There are finally important aspects on the follow-up of obscure findings as well as interesting information concerning the latest development in the management of early bronchial lesions, particularly photoirradiation by lasers via endoscopes.

This is a textbook which is not only a guide to the cytologic diagnosis of lung lesions but also a guideline to present and future development in the field of respiratory cytology.

Magnus Nasiell, M.D., F.I.A.C.

Preface

The role of cytology has been especially important in the recent progress in the field of lung cancer diagnosis. Due to the remarkable development of fiberoptic bronchoscopes and their accessories, in addition to improvement in percutaneous and transbronchial needle equipment and methods, it has become increasingly possible to obtain diagnostic cytologic materials directly from the lesion by a variety of methods, such as brushing cytology, TV brushing cytology, transbronchial aspiration cytology and percutaneous needle cytology and this has significantly increased the rate of diagnostic accuracy. Conventional sputum cytology in mass surveys has also become an essential method for the detection of X-ray-negative central type early stage lung cancer.

The rate of diagnostic accuracy of lung cancer at our institution has recently improved to 100% of central type cases and 99.8% in peripheral type cases. The main problem involving cytologic diagnosis is how to deal with suspicious cells, and there is also the question of arriving at the correct histologic diagnosis, which is important for the correct selection of therapeutic strategy and estimation of prognosis. This is frequently difficult to decide on the basis of the cytologic findings alone and it is generally necessary to include the results of clinical and laboratory examinations in order to obtain an accurate histologic diagnosis. It has been reported that diagnostic accuracy can be improved when the clinician obtains the cytology specimen and examines it himself. This exactly reflects the opinions of myself and the other authors, who are both clinicians and qualified cytologists. From this point of view, we have included the clinical aspects of cases in this book on cytology. In addition the type of cytological findings can differ even in the same case depending on the method by which the specimen was obtained, e.g. by sputum cytology as opposed to fresh cells from the lesion. Therefore the characteristics of specimens according to the method of harvesting have been included in the description.

The text offers a wide-ranging and thorough description of methods to obtain good specimens, which is of the essence in cytology, anatomy of the respiratory tract, the appearance of normal cells, cells of benign lesions, metaplastic cells, lung cancer cells and cytochemistry. In particular, in the chapter on squamous metaplasia a thorough description of the relationship with squamous cell carcinoma is provided which should be valuable in sputum cytology follow-up. Furthermore the chapter on cytochemistry shows how cytologic diagnostic methods and accuracy can go beyond the level of morphological evaluation alone by combination with morphological data.

This volume is intended for medical students, cytotechnicians and physicians specializing in cytology. As described it is intended to introduce clinical aspects to cytotechnicians and to describe to physicians methods to obtain specimens and understanding of the cytological findings.

In addition we would like to express our deep gratitude for the excellent and dedicated work of the cytotechnicians of Tokyo Medical College. In particular we would like to thank especially Mr. Hideaki Shima, C.T., I.A.C., who collected specimens and made the preparations for the photographs, and also (in alphabetical order) Toshiko Iida, C.T., I.A.C., Kimiko Saito, C.T., I.A.C., Michihiro Utsuki, C.T., I.A.C. and Akiko Yokoyama, C.T., I.A.C. for their continued high level of expertise. Without this background it would have been impossible for the authors to have been in a position to write this volume. We are also indebted to Associate Professor James Patrick Barron of St. Marianna University School of Medicine for his efforts in translating this volume from Japanese.

May 20, 1983

Harubumi Kato

Contents

I

Obtaining and Preparing Specimens

Methods to obtain specimens for the cytologic diagnosis of respiratory diseases differ according to the symptoms of the patient, the X-ray findings and the purpose of the examination. Table 1 shows the various types of methods that can be used to obtain specimens.

SPUTUM SPECIMENS

Sputum is a composite term for mixed secretions from the trachea, central bronchi, peripheral bronchi, alveoli containing cells exfoliated from their mucous membrane and from the lesion. The exfoliated cells are stained for cytologic diagnosis.

Early-morning sputum specimens yield the greatest amounts of diagnostic material. Material is obtained after gargling and rinsing the mouth to minimize

Table 1 Types of Specimens

1. Sputum
   1) Non-fixed sputum
   2) Saccomanno's method
   3) Mailing container method
      (Tokyo Medical College pooled sputum method)

2. Transfiberoptic bronchoscopic harvesting
   1) Brushing under endoscopic observation
   2) Under fluoroscopic TV monitoring
      a) brushing
      b) curettage
   3) Bronchial lavage
   4) Other methods

3. Needle cytology
   1) Percutaneous needle cytology
      a) Needle aspiration
      b) Needle with protrusions
      c) Other
   2) Transbronchial needle aspiration cytology
      a) Via the rigid bronchoscope
      b) Via the flexible fiberoptic bronchoscope
      c) Via the flexible fiberoptic bronchoscope
         under fluoroscopic TV monitoring

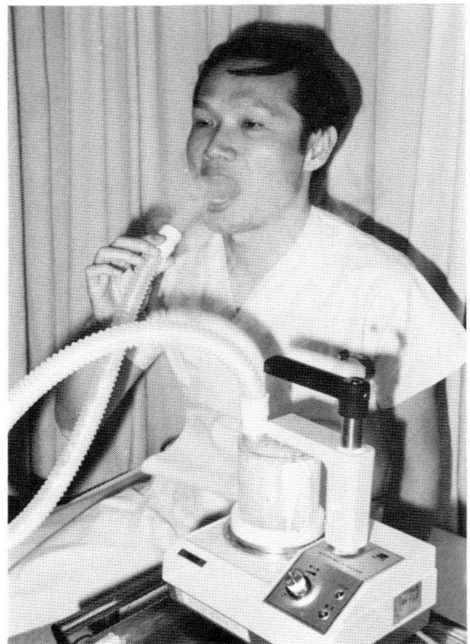

Fig. 1 Ultrasonic nebulizer to facilitate expectoration of sputum.

contamination by food residue and bacteria. Since the yield of diagnostic material is significantly greater with three specimens than with a single specimen, we recommend using specimens pooled over at least three days for cytologic studies including mass surveys (Hayata and Kato, 1979; Koss, 1979).

Many cases, especially those in mass surveys in which this method of examination is performed, do not complain of excessive amounts of sputum. Therefore, it is obviously difficult for such examinees to produce valid sputum specimens. In such cases, a mixture of 5% glycerine, 2% $NaHCO_3$ and 93% H_2O can be inspirated through a nebulizer (Fig. 1). Subsequently, the patient is instructed to take deep breaths, then to produce sputum. Repetition of this procedure can increase the yield of valid specimens. However, whereas this method is applicable in hospitalized examinees, outpatients using a mailing container generally do not have the necessary equipment (i.e. nebulizer). Such patients are instructed to breathe deeply over hot water or a humidifier at home.

Nonfixed Sputum

In this method the sputum of the inpatient or outpatient is placed in a Petri dish or test tube and immediately forwarded to the laboratory. To prevent

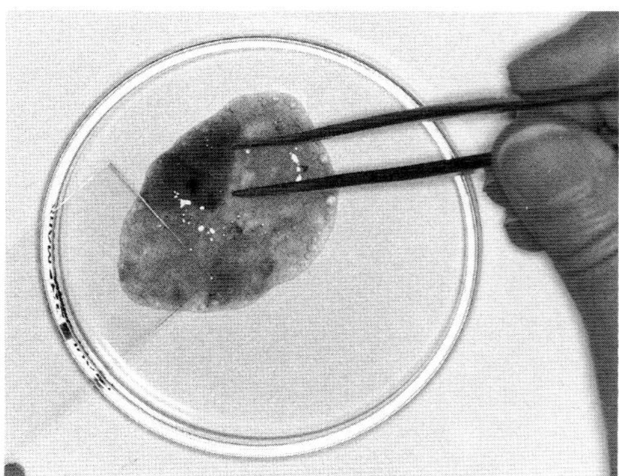

Fig. 2 Preparation of glass slide. Specimens are picked up with tweezers from the Petri dish. Rate of positive cancer cells is higher in the bloody areas.

Table 2 Comparison of mailing container (TMC) and Sacomanno methods

	Mailing container (TMC)	Saccomanno
Container size	9.5 x 6 x 1.6cm box	12 x 3.5 cm tube
Preservative/fixative	50% methyl alcohol, 1% timor	50% ethyl alcohol, carbowax
Specimen treatment	Smearing (Shibata, 1981)	Blending
Mucin	Remains	Disappears
Cell adhesion	Good	Poor, cells isolated
No. of specimens examined per day per screener	30	10
Strain on screener	Little	Eye fatigue
Positive diagnostic rate*	59.8%	59.0%
Other features	Suitable for mass surveys	Not suitable for mass surveys

* including peripheral lung cancers.

degeneration of cells in this method, smearing and staining must be performed quickly. This method yields highly stainable materials. Attention must be paid to which areas of the specimens most probably contain diagnostic materials. Cancer cells are often seen in bloody, brown areas of sputum (Fig. 2) (Koss, 1979; Takahashi, 1981). The specimen should be stained after fixing in 95% alcohol.

Mailing Container Method

This method is performed with specimens pooled over three days and, as can be seen in Table 2, yields a positive rate of 59.8%. However, because the examinee has to pool specimens for three days, the specimen return rate is low. As a result, patient education is extremely important. For this purpose we have published an educational pamphlet in Japanese for sputum cytology surveys originally developed by the Canadian Uranium Health and Safety Program at Elliot Lake Centre (Fig. 3) (Pearson et al.). The aim of the pamphlet is to increase awareness concerning the usefulness of sputum cytology examinations and to provide lucid and thorough instructions regarding sputum production. This method can be

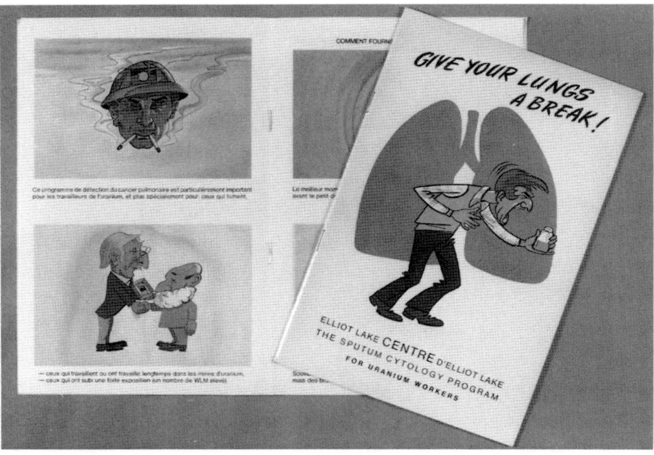

Fig. 3 An educational pamphlet for sputum cytology surveys. (Courtesy of Dr. F. G. Pearson, Elliot Lake Centre, Ontario, Canada)

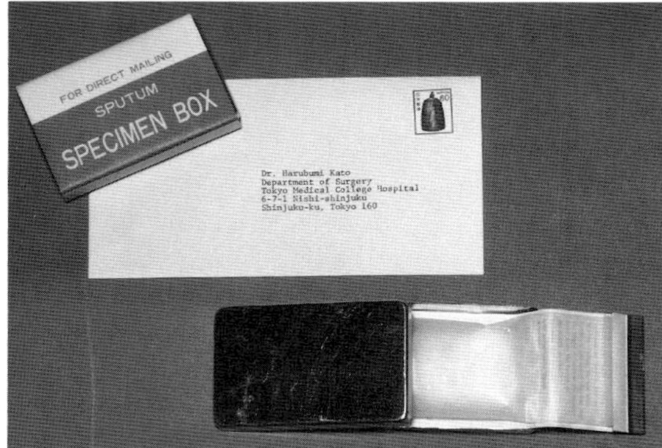

Fig. 4 Mailing container developed by Tokyo Medical College (TMC). A polyethylene pouch with fixative solution is contained in the aluminum box.

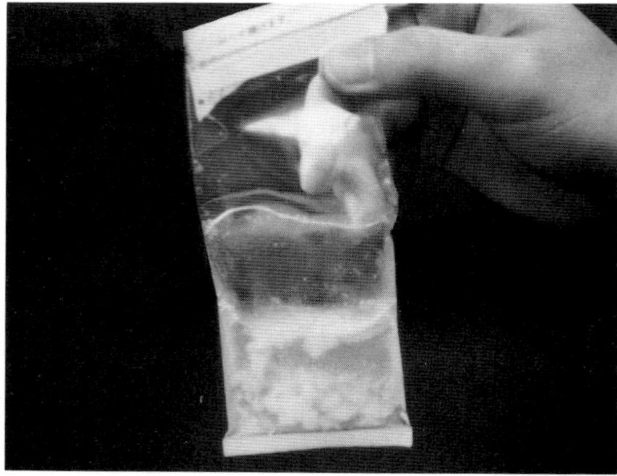

Fig. 5 Examinees cough out three-days' sputum into this polyethylene pouch of the TMC mailing container.

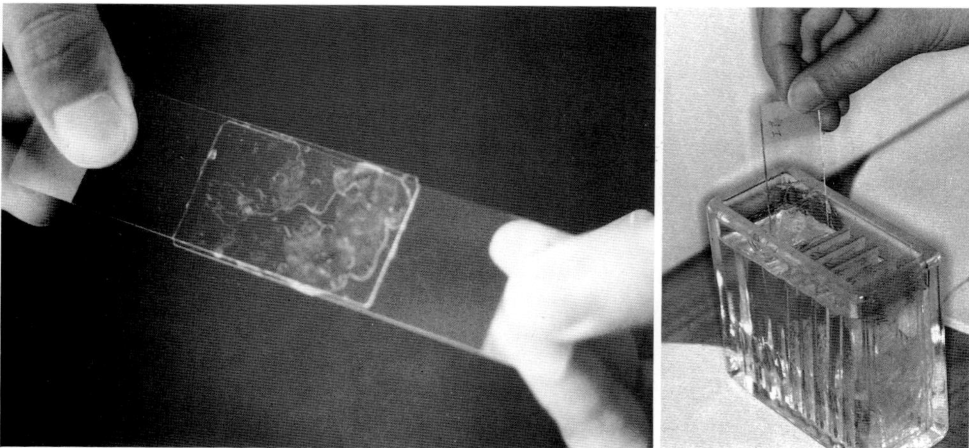

Fig. 6 The materials are picked up in the same way as shown in Figure 2 and sandwich-smeared as shown in this figure.

Fig. 7 The smeared glass slide is placed in a fixative solution of 95% alcohol or 10% formalin.

applied in mass surveys, for example in high-risk groups, with the subjects pooling daily specimens and then mailing the material in the container provided to the examination center (Fig. 4). The package developed by Tokyo Medical College for extensive surveys consists of a 9.5 × 6 × 1.6 cm aluminum container with a transparent, easily sealed 17 × 5.2 cm polyethylene pouch. The pouch contains a mixture of 9.9 ml of methyl alcohol and 0.1 ml of thymol as fixative and preservative. The subject cuts the corner of the polyethylene bag containing the fixative (Fig. 5), then produces sputum after cleansing the oral cavity and pharynx. After expectoration into the pouch, the subject seals the pouch by finger pressure, then shakes it thoroughly to obtain good contact with the preservative and fixative. The subject repeats the procedure for three days using the same pouch, then places the pouch in the aluminum box and mails it to the laboratory (Kato et al., 1982a). The pouch contents are poured on filter paper and the remaining materials are accumulated by a spatula and smeared on a glass slide. The material is sandwich smeared (Fig. 6) and fixed in 95% alcohol (Fig. 7). This process should be performed rapidly to prevent drying. Staining according to the Papanicolaou method (Papanicolaou, 1942) is then performed. The stainability of cells according to this method is generally good.

Saccomanno's Method

The subject expectorates sputum into a 12 cm long plastic tube with a diameter of 3.5 cm (Fig. 8) (Saccomanno et al., 1963). The tube is half filled with 50 ml of fixative consisting of 48 ml of 50% ethyl alcohol, 1 ml of 50% polyethylene glycol (Carbowax 1540) and 1 ml of ethyl alcohol containing 3 mg of Rifampin, and the subject is instructed to shake the tube well to mix the contents thoroughly. The contents of the tube are transferred to a 50 ml centrifuge tube.

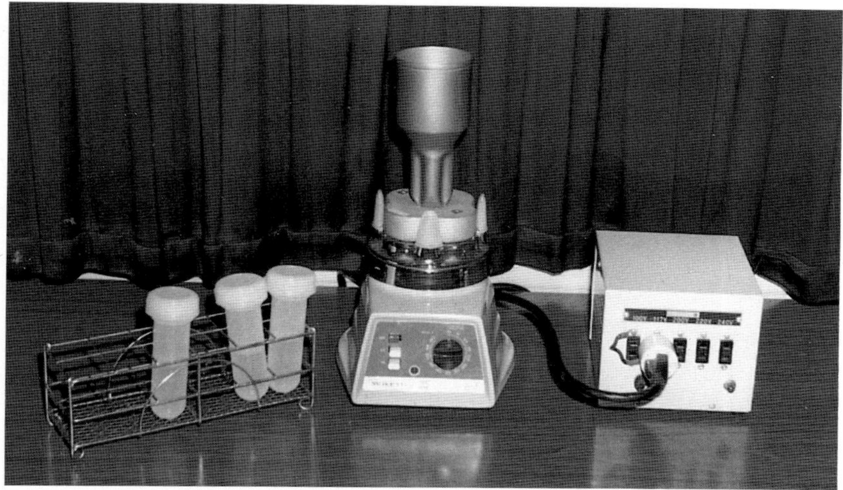

Fig. 8 Saccomanno's container and blender. Examinees cough out three-days' sputum into a plastic tube. The material is blended to liquify the mucous fibers.

If necessary, the contents of the tube are increased by 50% ethanol. The material is then transferred to a blender (See Fig. 8) for 3 to 4 seconds of high-speed blending (22,000 rpm). The mixture is then observed, and if still granular, it is blended again for 2 to 3 seconds until it reaches a cloudy, liquid, homogeneous state. The material is then transferred to a 50 ml glass or plastic tube and centrifuged for 15 minutes at 1,500 rpm. After removal of the supernatants the sediment is smeared on glass slides. Slides prepared by this method are generally replete with material, and cells often appear isolated as a result of the blending process.

Comparison of Mailing Container Method and Saccomanno's Method

Table 2 shows the differences between these two methods in regard to the detection of cancer cells, determination of the degree of degeneration of cancer cells, the number of specimens that can be examined per day by a single cyto-technician and features of such cells that can be distinguished. We find that the mailing container method allows a greater number of specimens to be examined per day by each investigator (Figures 9–11).

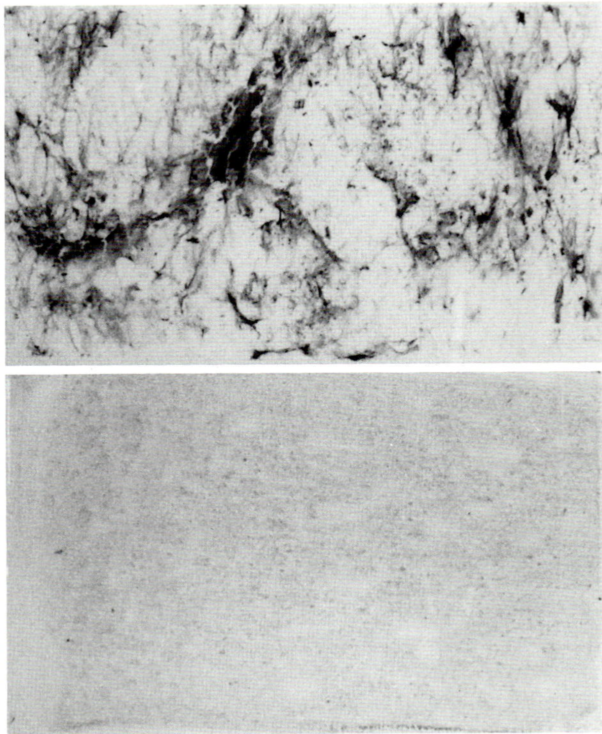

Fig. 9 Differences in the smears prepared by the TMC (top) and the Saccomanno method (bottom).

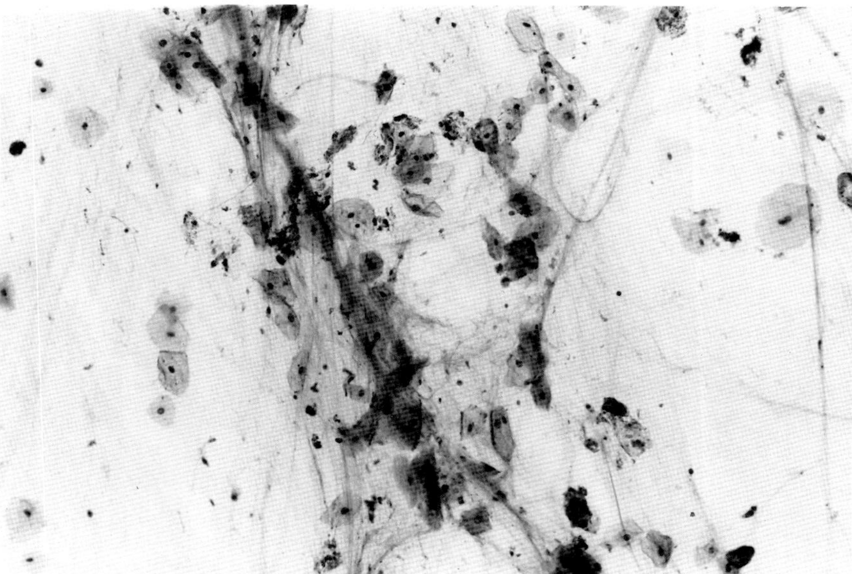

Fig. 10 TMC smear preparation. This specimen shows the same features as routine clinical laboratory sputum smear preparations. Cellular adherence is preserved. (× 100: Magnifications in this book are given as the total overall magnification, i.e. enlargement of the photograph multiplied by the magnification of the objective lens. Pap.)

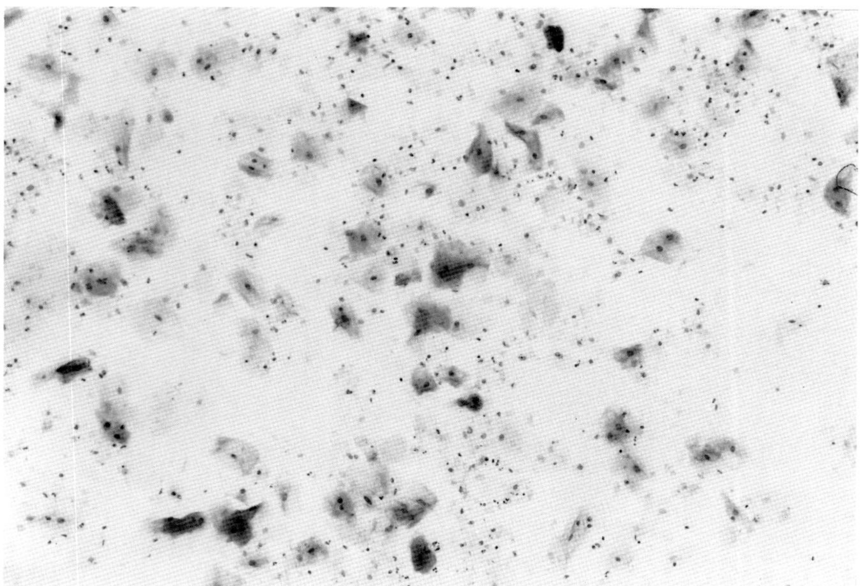

Fig. 11 Saccomanno preparation. This method has the advantage of yielding a larger rate of cells per smear preparation although the nature of the method of preparation, i.e. blending in a mixer, can cause artificial changes in the cells in the smear. (×100, **Pap.**)

TRANSFIBEROPTIC BRONCHOSCOPIC HARVESTING

With the development of the fiberoptic bronchoscope (Ikeda, 1974), the ability to definitively diagnose lung cancer has increased remarkably. The fiberoptic bronchoscope enables not only visualization of central type lung cancer lesions but also histologic biopsy, cytologic brushing and curettage of peripheral lesions under X-ray fluorography.

Before performing fiberoptic bronchoscopy, the patient's condition is checked. Fifteen minutes before the procedure is begun, atropine sulfate is administered intramuscularly to minimize bronchial secretions. The local anesthetic spray is 4% lidocaine. After ascertaining that the patient has responded normally to the lidocaine test, the nasal lumen, base of the tongue, pharynx and larynx are sprayed with the anesthetic via a Jackson spray to obtain superficial anesthesia (Fig. 12). The fiberoptic bronchoscope can then be inserted either transnasally or transorally.

The transnasal method minimizes stimulation of the pharynx, thereby reducing the pharyngeal reflex and allowing the amount of anesthesia to be kept to a minimum, and is also helpful in the detection of nasopharyngeal tumors (Fig. 13).

In cases of hypertrophic sinusitis, deformity of the middle meatus or nasal polyp, in which nasal insertion is impossible, the transoral route is the insertion route of choice. The amount of anesthetic required in the latter case is about three times more than is required in the former. The transoral route involves the risk of damage to the instrument if the patient bites it; therefore, a mouthpiece must be put in place.

The stability of the fiberoptic bronchoscope is enhanced by transnasal insertion. We find that a smooth procedure can generally be performed after

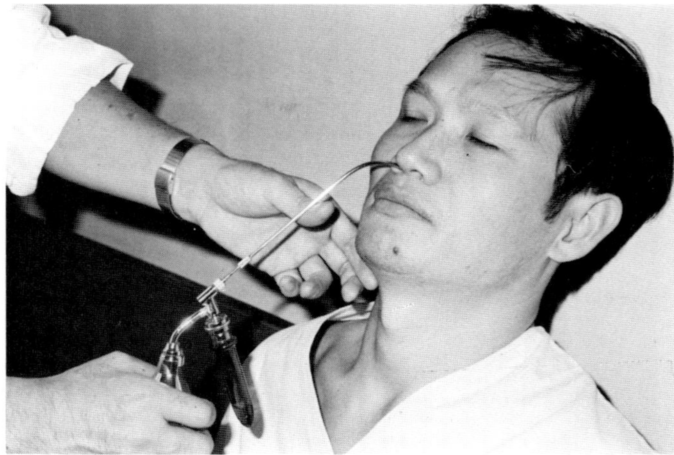

Fig. 12 Local anesthesia is performed with 5—10 cc of 4% lidocaine. The nasal lumen and the base of the tongue, pharynx and larynx are sprayed with a Jackson spray.

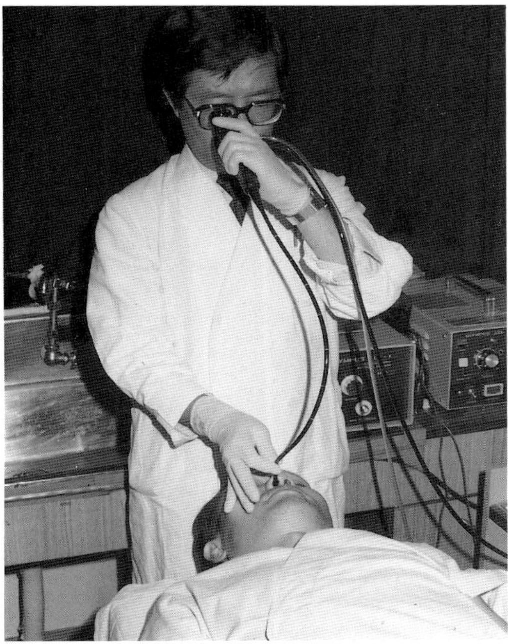

Fig. 13 Transnasal insertion of the fiberoptic bronchoscope.

squirting 1 ml of 2—4% lidocaine jelly via a small disposable conical cap into the nasal lumen along the insertion route. After insertion, the mouth is closed and care is always exercised to ensure that the tip of the instrument is maintained in the center of the lumen as it is advanced. Once the tip reaches the larynx, the patient is asked to breathe deeply, and the tip of the fiberoptic bronchoscope is advanced gently between the vocal cords into the trachea, through the bronchus and up to the lesion.

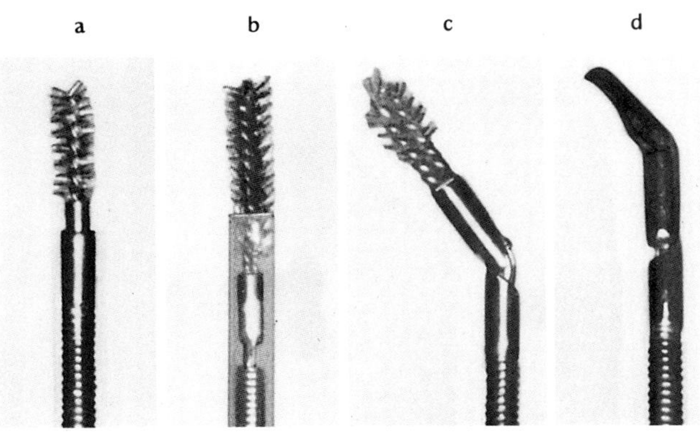

Fig. 14 Cytology brushes and curette. The jointed instruments (c and d) simplify the procedure and improve accuracy in cases of lesions located in sites difficult to reach. These are generally employed under X-ray monitoring.
(a)   Standard cytology brush.
(b)   Cytology brush with sheath which is used to avoid contamination.
(c)   Double-joint cytology brush.
(d)   Double-joint curette.

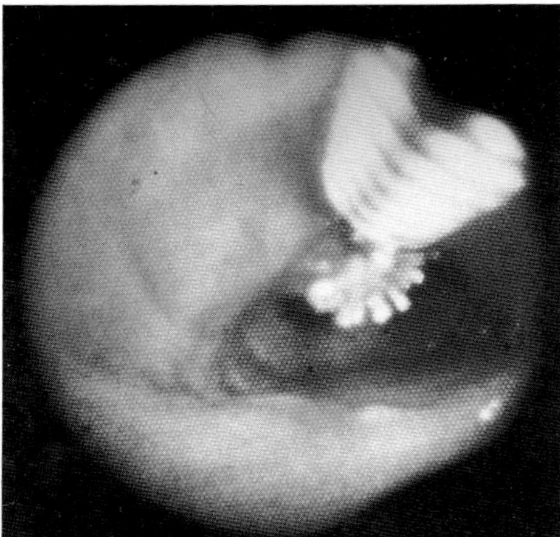

Fig. 15 Obtaining a brushing cytology specimen from the middle lobe bronchus.

Brushing Under Endoscopic Visualization

The various fiberoptic bronchoscopes that are available have been designed for use in different situations. The standard instrument has a diameter of about 5.3 mm, but the diameter can vary from 4.4 to 5.9 mm. The thinnest models allow visualization of subsubsegmental bronchi.

In this method, the tumor is examined visually, then cells are obtained from the tumor surface by means of a plastic brush at the end of a spiral stainless steel wire. The authors usually use BC-5C or BC-9C brushes (Olympus Optical Co.) (Fig. 14). The brush is inserted through the instrumentation channel of the fiberoptic bronchoscope and rubbed several times against the target surface (Fig. 15). To prevent dissemination of cells or contamination it is best to use a brush with a sheath. In cases of tumors accompanied by necrosis, it is important to avoid necrotic areas when brushing. Cells that adhere to the brush are smeared with a circular motion on a glass slide over an area 2 cm in diameter (Fig. 16). The

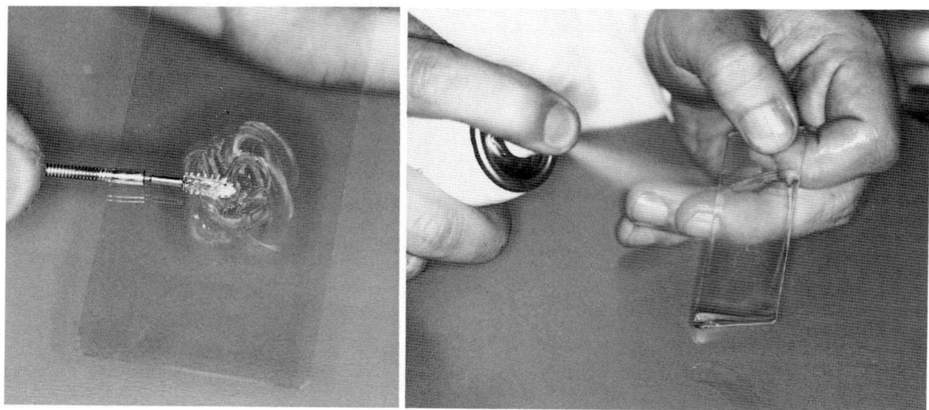

Fig. 16 The brushing specimen is smeared on a glass slide immediately after brushing.

Fig. 17 The smeared specimen is immediately fixed with isopropyl alcohol spray to avoid cellular degeneration.

material is not spread over too wide an area to prevent drying of the specimen and to facilitate rapid screening. Fixing is performed immediately after smearing, either by dipping in, or spraying with 95% alcohol (Fig. 17). Unless fixing is performed rapidly, morphologic changes will occur as a result of drying.

This method is extremely effective, not only for definitive diagnosis but also for determining the extent of invasion. When performing brushing of several sites, care should be taken to avoid contamination. In such cases, the need for a separate brush with its own cover for each brushing site is obvious. This method has no intrinsic complications. Although material can also be obtained by curettage, brushes have been shown to provide satisfactory results.

Brushing Under X-ray Television Monitoring

Peripheral lung cancer lesions are frequently difficult to visualize by fiberoptic bronchoscopy. In such cases, biopsy forceps, a brush or a curette is inserted up to the lesion under X-ray fluoroscopic guidance to obtain material for cytologic diagnosis (Hattori et al., 1964, 1965; Tsuboi, 1970). The patient is prepared in the same way as for routine fiberoptic bronchoscopy, with local anesthesia performed in the X-ray fluoroscopy room. The tip of the fiberoptic bronchoscope is inserted into the bronchus in which the lesion is thought to be located. The relative locations of the fiberoptic bronchoscope tip and the lesion are then confirmed on an X-ray television screen, and a brush or double-jointed curette is inserted until the X-ray television screen shows that it protrudes from the tip of the fiberoptic bronchoscope (Fig. 18). The brush or curette is next inserted

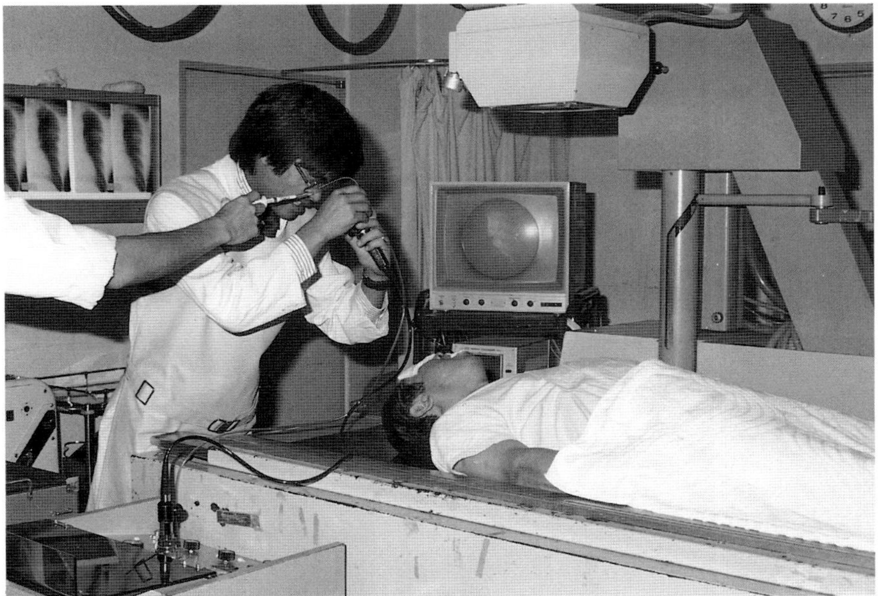

Fig. 18 TV-brushing. The brushing technique is performed by fiberoptic bronchoscopy under X-ray TV monitoring.

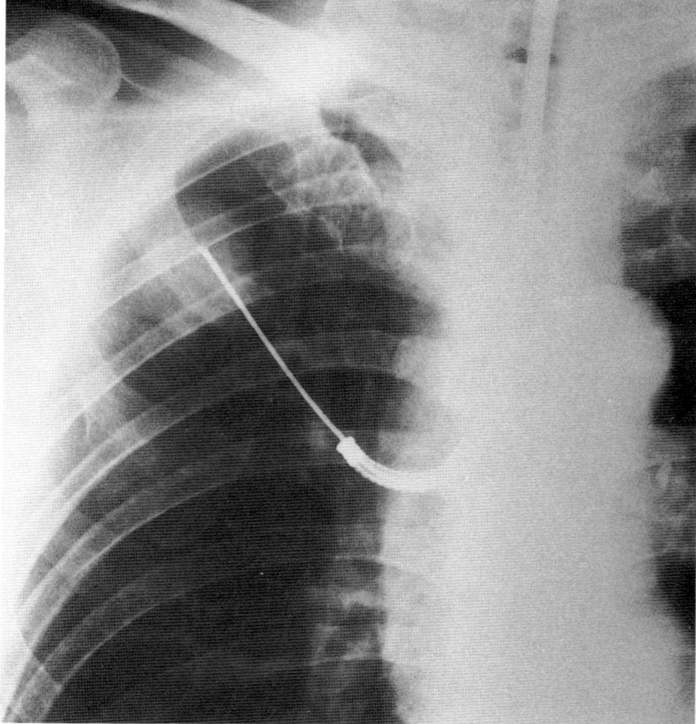

Fig. 19 TV-brushing under X-ray TV monitoring.

toward the lesion under X-ray television guidance (Fig. 19). To negotiate peripheral bronchial bifurcations, which anatomically present problems for insertion, a double-jointed brush or curette is used. Such an accessory permits control of the angle of the brush or curette to permit selective insertion into the target bronchus. When the brush or curette reaches the lesion, further insertion is prevented by the resistance of the lesion, and this sensation indicates the site to be curetted or brushed. After the site has been rubbed several times, the tip of the brush or curette is retracted into the sheath, and withdrawn through the instrumentation channel. After withdrawal, the harvested material is smeared and immediately fixed as explained above. This method has caused no complications.

Bronchial Lavage

In cases in which sputum cytology examination reveals malignant cells but the chest X-ray film shows no abnormalities, fiberoptic bronchoscopy is immediately performed. However, if no abnormal findings are recognized endoscopically, bronchial lavage is indicated to localize the lesion (Koss, 1979; Kato et al., 1982b). In this method, the bronchi in the right and left lungs are first washed individually; then each segmental bronchus from B_1 to B_{10} in both lungs is washed selectively, and the washing fluid is retrieved and sealed in separate

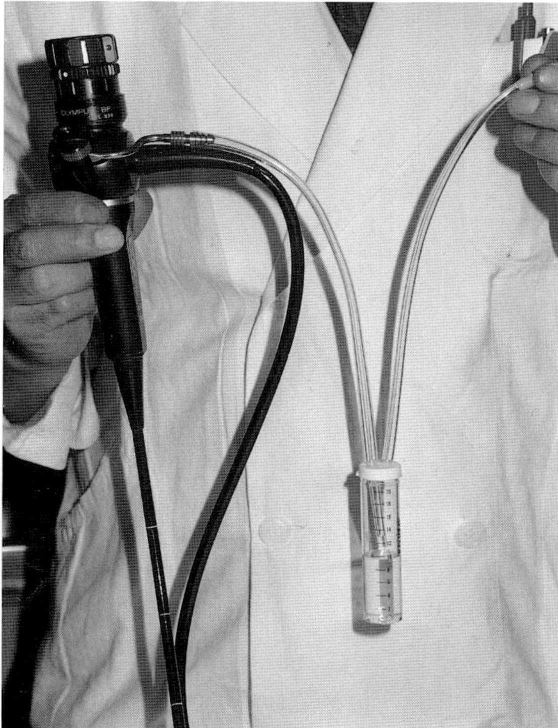

Fig. 20 Container for bronchial washing cytology. The collection vessel is attached to the suction channel of the fiberoptic bronchoscope.

containers. A container with 5 ml of 50% alcohol solution should be used to prevent cellular degeneration (Ono et al., 1982). The cells contained in the fluid are then examined. For washing of each segmental bronchus, 10 ml of physiologic saline is instilled via a washing catheter inserted through the instrumentation channel, and the patient is instructed to breathe out as the washing fluid is aspirated via the instrumentation channel of the fiberoptic bronchoscope. The collection vessel is attached to the instrumentation channel (Fig. 20). Since the bronchial lavage method involves retrieval of washings from different bronchi through the same instrumentation channel, there is often a risk of contamination. Therefore, after washing each segmental bronchus, the fiberoptic bronchoscope must be removed and the instrumentation channel should be flushed with sterilizing disinfectant. For this procedure, we employ chlorhexidine solution.

Washings from each segmental bronchus are placed in clearly marked tubes and sent immediately to the cytology laboratory, where they are centrifuged at 1,500 rpm for 15 minutes. The supernatant is discarded, and the sediment is transferred to a glass slide using a pipette. Another slide is placed on the glass slide to obtain two smears, then the smears are fixed again in 95% alcohol or 10% formalin. This method is particularly useful in the localization of peripheral occult lung cancer.

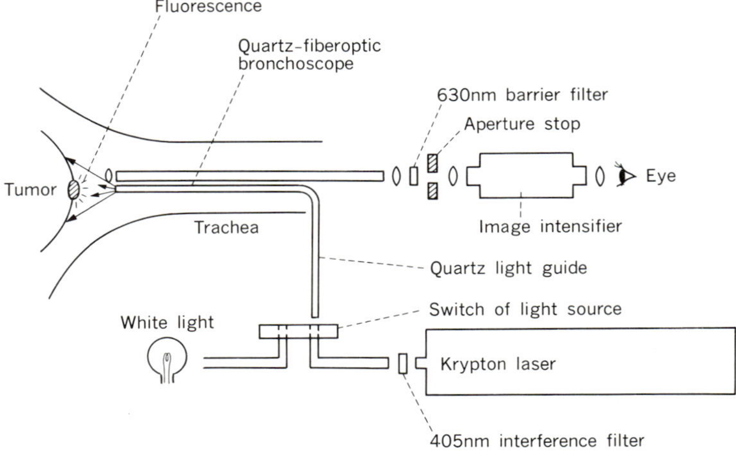

Fig. 21 Schema of diagnostic apparatus. A krypton ion laser is used as a light source. The laser beam is guided through the instrumentation channel of the fiberoptic bronchoscope via 400 μ quartz fiber. The specific fluorescence of hematoporphyrin derivative from the tumor focus is observed through the image intensifier which gives a luminous gain of x 30,000.

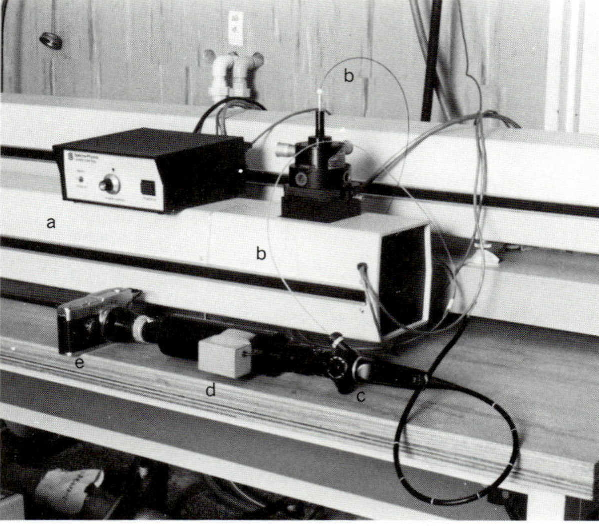

Fig. 22 Diagnostic apparatus.
(a)   Krypton ion laser.
(b)   Quartz fiber.
(c)   Fiberoptic bronchoscope.
(d)   Image intensifier.
(e)   Camera.

Other Methods

Laser photoradiation

Cases of occult lung cancer are generally at an extremely early stage, for example, carcinoma in situ, and in such cases mucosal changes are macroscopically not recognizable. Localization of such cancers by conventional diagnostic techniques borders on the impossible. The laser photoradiation method with a hematoporphyrin derivative (Figs. 21 and 22) seems potentially useful in the localization and

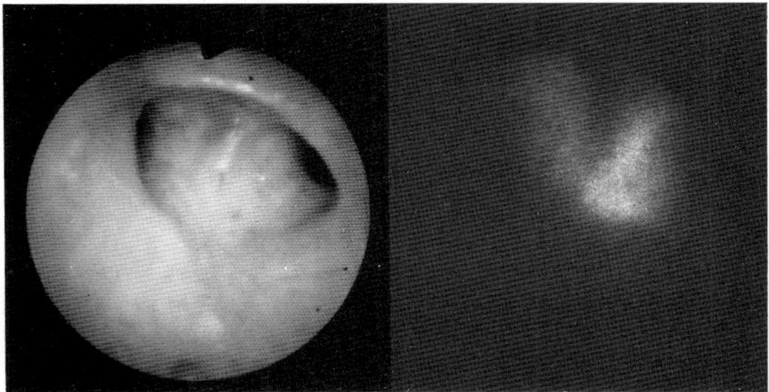

a   b

Fig. 23 (a) Slight thickness at the bifurcation of the segmental bronchi in the right upper lobe
bronchus is observed.
(b)   Slight fluorescence is seen at a site corresponding to the thickness. The results of brushing
cytology strongly suggested squamous cell carcinoma.

diagnosis of such cases originating in larger bronchi although further studies are required to fully clarify the role of this technique. Hematoporphyrin derivative has been shown to be retained longer by malignant tissue than by normal tissue (Profio and Doiron, 1977; Kinsey et al., 1978; Doiron et al., 1979; Kato et al., 1981a; Hayata et al., 1982a, b). It also has the interesting characteristics of red light fluorescence on stimulation by violet light (Fig. 23). Since fluorescence is suggestive of malignancy, such areas are carefully brushed for morphologic examination using the instrumentation and methodology described previously.

Dye-spraying method

Several dyes have been used for the localization of cancerous lesions, especially in the alimentary tract. Such dyes include toluidine blue (Endo et al., 1972; Yoshida, 1981), Lugol, toluidine blue-iodine, indigocarmine, Congo red and fluorescence dyes (Takemoto et al., 1976). Macroscopic diagnosis is made on the basis of the specific pattern of staining of the specimen after the dye is sprayed.

NEEDLE CYTOLOGY SPECIMENS

Needle biopsy of the lung has a history of over a century. The first report was in 1883 by Leyden, who performed the procedure for bacteriologic diagnosis of pneumonia. The report by Ménétrier on the use of this method for the diagnosis of lung cancer in 1886 was followed by many others, but this method failed to gain widespread recognition because of associated complications. In 1930, Martin and Ellis reported their results with the procedure using a thin needle; this report was followed by those of Craver and Binkley (1939) and Gledhill et al. (1949) on their experience with the method in the diagnosis of lung tumors.

This method became more widely employed in the 1960s through the development of the X-ray image-enhanced television screen and the pioneering work of Sönderström (1966), Dahlgren (1967), Sinner (1973) and Nordenström (1975) in Sweden. In Japan, the first report was made by Kawai and Katsuki in

1956; this report was followed by the development of needles by Hayata and coworkers (1973) and by Okamoto and his colleagues (1974).

Material for the cytologic diagnosis of lung cancer can be obtained by needles inserted either percutaneously or transbronchially.

Percutaneous Route

This method can be broken down into two basic methods: needle aspiration cytology and the use of a needle with fine protrusions to which cells adhere.

Aspiration method

For this procedure, a needle having a length of 9 to 16 cm and an outer diameter of 0.6 to 1.2 mm is generally used. However, there is no need to be overly concerned about precise needle dimensions; the needle must simply be long enough to reach the lesion and allow 23- or 21-gauge aspiration (Fig. 24) (Kato and Ono, 1982).

The point in the chest wall closest to the lesion is first determined on the basis of the posteroanterior and lateral chest X-ray films to obtain the shortest possible puncture route. Before the procedure, 20 mg of hydroxyzine hydrochloride is injected intramuscularly after the patient's condition has been checked. It is also important to explain the procedure to the patient in detail to prevent undue worry and stress as well as to obtain full cooperation. The procedure is performed in the X-ray television room. The patient is asked to lie on the examination table, and his or her position is determined according to the site of the lesion. Care is then exercised to obtain sufficient local invasive anesthesia of the pleura using 0.5 −1.0% lidocaine. Puncture is usually performed under X-ray television guidance, but if the lesion is large and near the chest wall, this may not be necessary. The patient is instructed to breathe regularly. Recognizable movement of the lesion by the tip of the needle confirms that the needle has reached the lesion. Once the

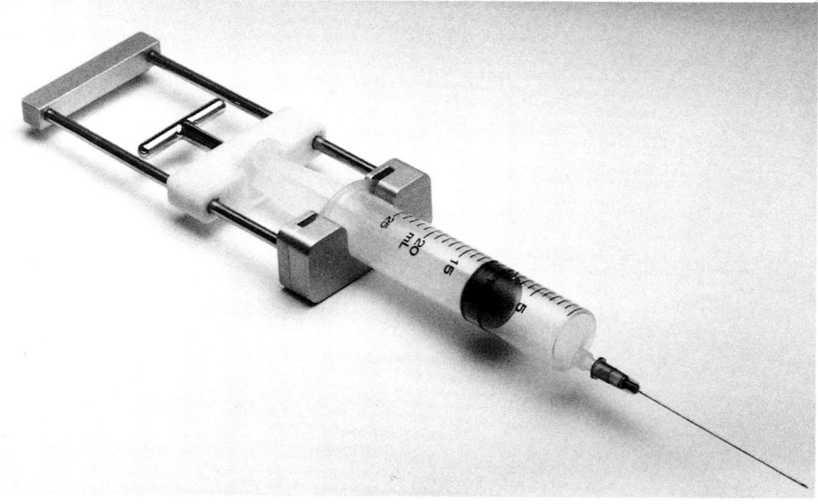

Fig. 24 Syringe and holder for aspiration cytology.

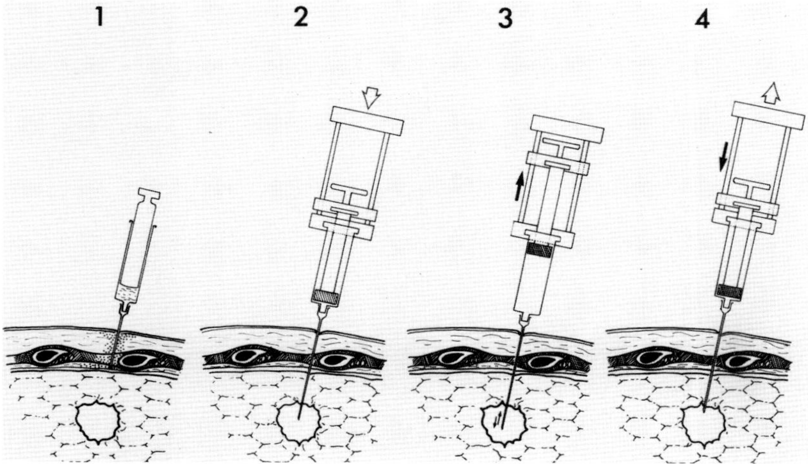

Fig. 25 Schema of aspiration procedure.
(1)   Skin, muscle and pleura are anesthesized with 1% lidocaine.
(2)   Puncture of the tumor is performed under TV monitoring.
(3)   Aspiration is performed moving the needle slightly backwards and forwards in the tumor.
(4)   After aspiration is completed, the syringe plunger is returned to a neutral position and the needle is removed from the chest wall.

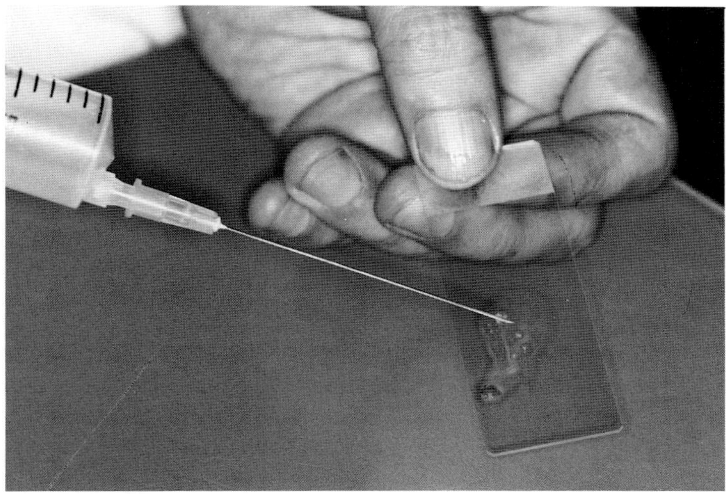

Fig. 26 The aspirated material in the needle is expelled onto a glass slide. It must be fixed immediately to avoid cellular degeneration.

lesion has been penetrated, a 20-ml disposable syringe is attached, and aspiration is performed. During aspiration, the tip of the needle is moved slightly, returned to a neutral position and then the needle is removed from the chest wall (Fig. 25). After removal, the syringe is filled with air to expel the material in the needle onto a glass slide for immediate fixation (Fig. 26). Aspiration is simplified if a holder such as that shown in Figure 24 is used. It is also important to confirm that the tip of the needle is actually in the lesion during the aspiration procedure and to remember that sudden aspiration when the tip is in the parenchyma of the lung involves the risk of pulmonary embolism.

Fixation is performed with 95% alcohol or 10% formalin, or by spraying with isopropyl alcohol as described in the previous section, taking care to prevent drying of the specimen. Usually, Papanicolaou staining and May-Giemsa staining are performed.

Needle with fine protrusions

This procedure employs a set of two needles: an outer sheath and an inner needle with many fine protrusions to which cells adhere. There are two versions of this needle, which was developed at the Department of Surgery of Tokyo Medical College. The shorter needle was developed in 1967 and the longer one in 1978. The outer diameters of the outer needles in the two versions are the same (1 mm), but the lengths are different, 80 and 150 mm. Accordingly, the lengths of the inner needles differ, 120 and 190 mm. The protrusions extend 20 mm from the tip (Fig. 27) (Kato et al., 1982b). To permit simple evaluation of the depth to which the needle has been inserted, the outer needle has marks at centimeter intervals from the tip.

The clinical procedure is almost exactly the same as that described in the previous section for aspiration cytology (Fig. 28). The only difference is that in this method, great care is exercised to prevent the tip of the outer needle from

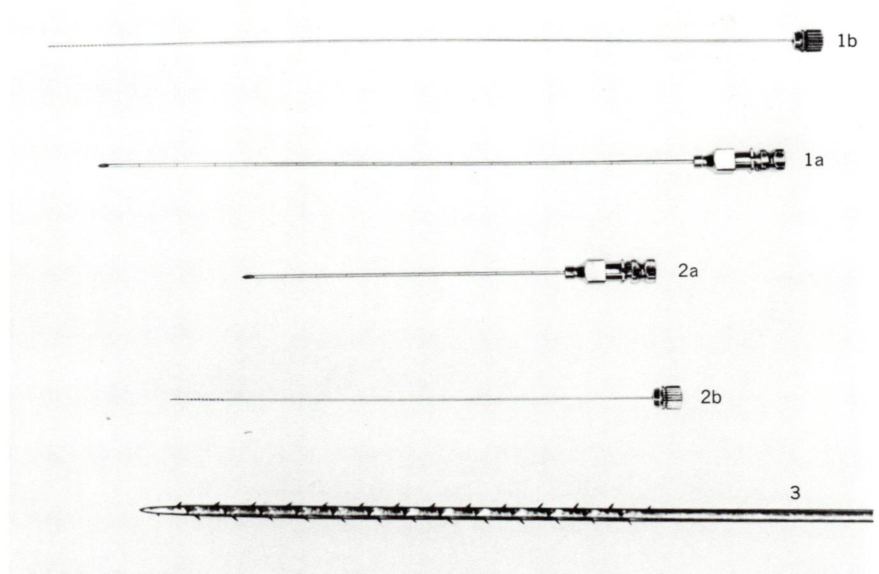

Fig. 27 TMC needles
(1a)   The outer needle is 1.0mm in diameter and 150mm in length.
(1b)   The inner needle is 190mm in length with protrusions 20mm from the tip.
(2a)   The outer needle is 1.0mm in diameter and 80mm in length.
(2b)   The inner needle is 120mm in length with protrusions 20mm from the tip.
(3)   Magnification of the tip of the inner needle.
(Takei Co., Ltd., Tokyo)

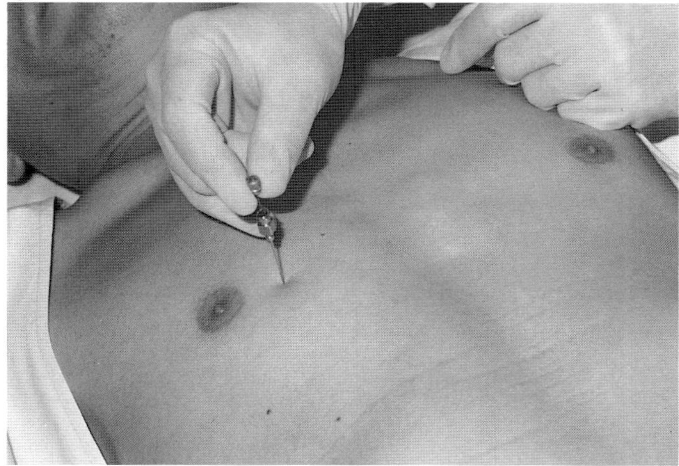

Fig. 28 TMC-needle method. Material is obtained by rotating the inner needle in the tumor.

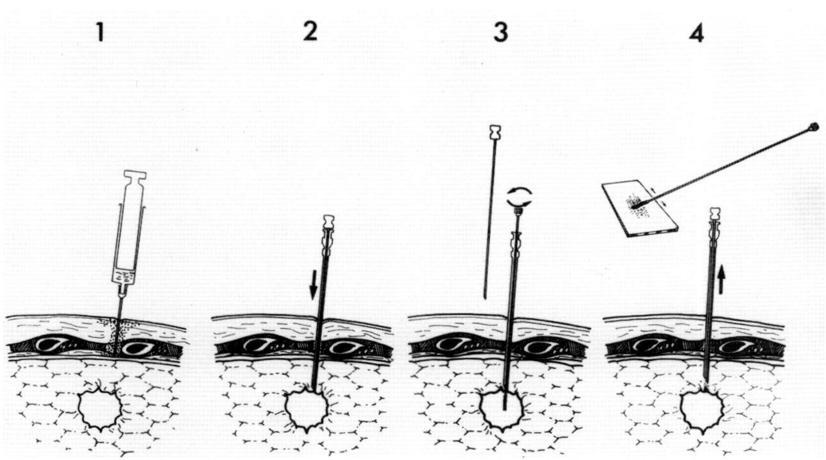

Fig. 29 Schema of the TMC-needle technique.
(1)   Skin, muscle and pleura are anesthesized with 1% lidocaine.
(2)   Puncture of chest wall at a site close to the tumor is performed under X-ray TV monitoring.
(3)   The inner needle with protrusions is inserted into the tumor through the outer needle and is rotated several times.
(4)   The inner needle is removed from the tumor through the outer needle and the specimen is smeared on the glass slide and fixed immediately.

actually puncturing the lesion so that malignant cells are not disseminated along the needle tract. Therefore, in this method the outer needle is brought up to just in front of the lesion, and the inner needle is inserted into the lesion to harvest the cell specimens (Fig. 29) (Kato et al., 1980a). It is thus obvious that posteroanterior and lateral chest X-ray films must be evaluated carefully before the procedure is begun. It is also important to rotate the inner needle two or three times once it has been inserted inside the lesion to obtain adhesion of sufficient material (Fig. 30). The inner needle is then removed, and its contents are smeared on a glass slide. After this procedure has been repeated four or five times with

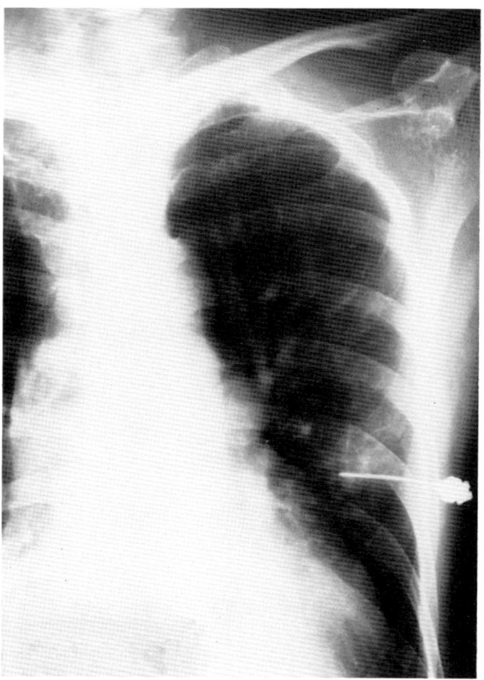

Fig. 30 X-ray TV findings during the percutaneous needle technique.

new inner needles, the outer needle is removed. When inserting the outer needle, an indwelling mandrin is used to prevent skin, muscle and pleura from entering the needle lumen. One of the advantages of this method is that even with very hard lesions, such as hamartomas and fibrous mesotheliomas, sufficient material can be obtained to allow definitive diagnosis. Smearing and fixation as described above are immediately performed.

Other methods

Many different types of needles have been developed. The needle developed by Nordenström (1975) consists of an outer needle having a length of 19.5 cm engraved with a screwlike groove designed to receive the specimen as the needle is rotated in the lesion. The needle developed by Franzén for examination of the prostate is 22 cm long with an external diameter of 0.6 mm. Other needles have been designed for histologic biopsy but involve higher complication rates.

Table 3 Complications of percutaneous needle cytology

No. of procedures: 1,246
Period: May 1967 — July 1981

	No. of cases	Percentage
Pneumothorax	67	5.4%
Bloody sputum	41	3.3
Hemoptysis	2	0.2
Shock	2	0.2
Pyothorax	1	0.08
Implantation	1	0.08
	114	9.14%

Complications

A total of 1,246 needle cytology procedures were carried out at the Department of Surgery of Tokyo Medical College between May 1967 and July 1981. Complications occurred in 9.14% of cases. As is shown in Table 3, the most frequently observed complication was pneumothorax, followed by bloody sputum, and there was one case of implantation of malignant cells in the needle tract. Only two cases of pneumothorax necessitated the insertion of a drain; the other 65 cases were relatively mild. Although implantation of malignant cells is an extremely rare complication, it is one that deserves careful consideration. In our case, the patient presented with cough, and a coin lesion 2 cm in diameter was recognized in the right middle lung field. Repeated sputum cytology examinations and fiberoptic bronchoscopic brushing under X-ray television guidance failed to yield a diagnosis. Percutaneous needle biopsy was therefore performed via the anterior thoracic wall, and a definitive diagnosis of adenocarcinoma was made, on the basis of which right middle and upper bilobectomy was performed. The tumor had a diameter of 2.5 cm, and there was no pleural adhesion or effusion, nor was there pleural invasion. The procedure was therefore considered curative. The histologic diagnosis of the resected specimen was poorly differentiated adenocarcinoma. The patient complained of anterior chest wall pain 19 months after lobectomy. The site of the small protrusion corresponded to that of the puncture, and extirpation of the tumor revealed that it was a metastatic lesion.

Tumors deriving from implantation in the needle tract have been reported by many investigators (Ochsner et al., 1947; Dutra and Geraci, 1954; Aronovitch et al., 1963; Wolinsky and Lishner, 1969; Berger et al., 1972; Nordenström and Dahlgren, 1966; Ichiba et al., 1975; Sinner, 1976; King et al., 1976), but there is no published report suggesting that the incidence of this complication is high. However, although the incidence is low, this complication deserves serious consideration, and the authors have expended considerable effort to prevent its occurrence, especially after encountering this single case. The cause of this complication can be considered to be insertion of the outer needle into the lesion, with material detaching as the needle is withdrawn and remaining in the needle tract in the thoracic wall. Therefore, the ideal solution is to avoid contact between the outer needle and the lesion and to make sure that only the inner needle penetrates the lesion when collecting specimens. Although this precaution may be difficult to put into practice, one must try as hard as possible to perform the·procedure in this ideal fashion.

There have been eight cases in the literature of death after needle biopsy (Woolf, 1954; Lauby et al., 1965; Adamson and Bates, 1967; Meyer et al., 1970; Johnsson and Schnürer, 1971; Westcott, 1973); in all eight cases, thick needles (2.2 to 2.5 mm) were used. There have been no reports of death after use of a fine needle (1 mm).

The most frequent complication was pneumothorax, which can be prevented to some degree by sufficient care. The incidence of pneumothorax is generally low in the hands of experienced clinicians making single quick punctures. Factors that increase the risk of pneumothorax include advanced age, deep punctures and concurrent chronic lung diseases.

Aspiration Cytology Via The Bronchoscope

Via the rigid bronchoscope

This technique was first reported by Versteegh and Swierenga in 1963, and there have been subsequent reports by Grunze (1966), Pichlmaier et al. (1970), Sawada et al. (1971), Törzsök (1975), Hiddink and Lopes Cardozo (1977), Sato et al. (1977) and Ballin (1977). These investigators performed the procedure in cases of lung tumors or to determine metastasis to bronchial bifurcation lymph nodes using rigid bronchoscopes.

However, since this procedure is performed using rigid bronchoscopes, it has disadvantages, including work-up before the procedure, pain and discomfort experienced by the patient and the long time that the procedure takes. In this method a long needle is inserted, and the specimen is smeared on glass slides, fixed and stained.

Via the fiberoptic bronchoscope

This method and the devices that make it possible were developed by some of the authors (H.K., J.O., C.K., Y.H.) and their colleagues in 1977 (Kato et al., 1978a, 1980a, b). The retractable needle used in this procedure is at the tip of a 110 cm long flexible catheter encased by a stainless steel coil having an outer diameter of 1.7 mm (Fig. 31). There are two versions of the retractable needle. One has a tip length of 8 mm when fully extended and an outer diameter of 0.6 mm; the other has a length of 10 mm and an outer diameter of 0.8 mm (Fig. 32). The authors have also developed a longer needle with an additional lateral opening (Fig. 33). Extension or retraction of the needle within its sheath at the tip can be controlled by the control unit outside the fiberoptic bronchoscope.

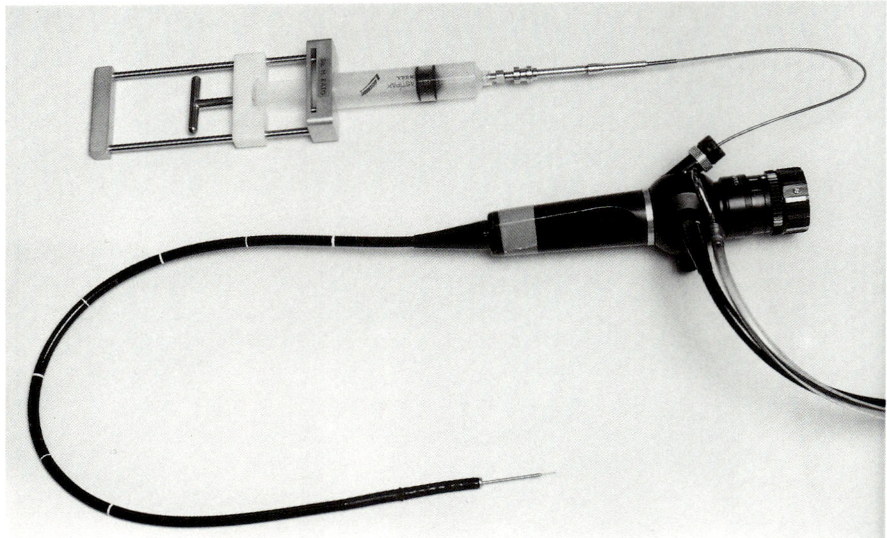

Fig. 31 TMC flexible aspiration cytology via the needle designed for use with the fiberoptic bronchoscope. (Olympus Co.)

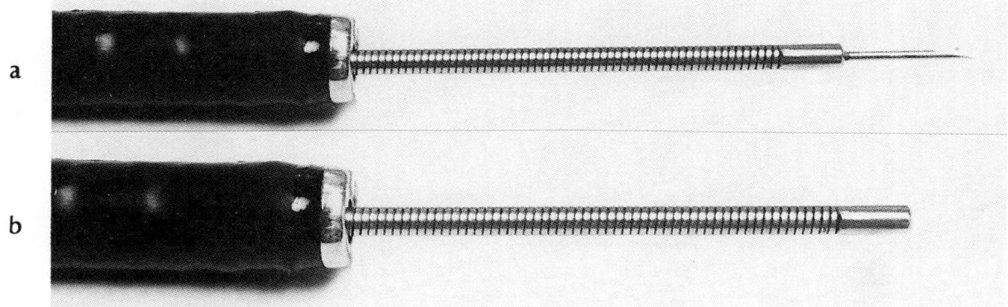

Fig. 32 Magnification of the tip of the TMC flexible needle.
(a) Needle extended from tip.
(b) Needle retracted inside tip.

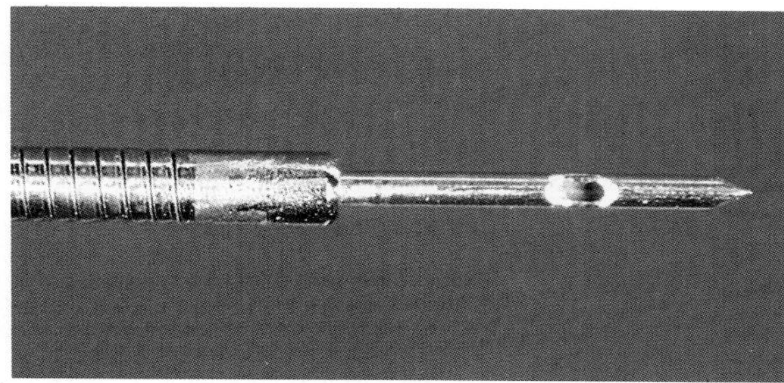

Fig. 33 Needle with openings at the tip and side obtains greater amount of diagnostic material.

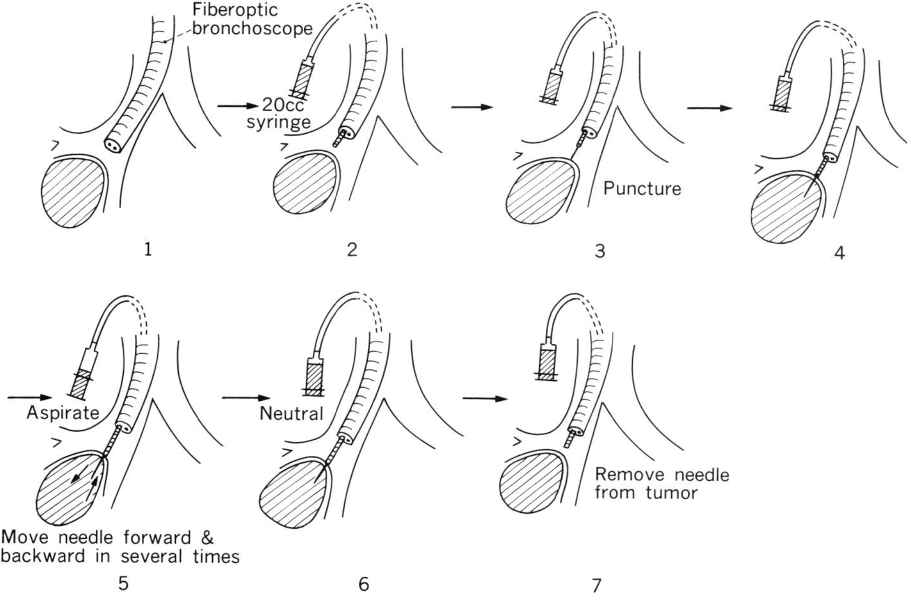

Fig. 34 Schema of the transbronchial needle aspiration cytology (TBAC) procedure. Previously published in Jap. J. Clin. Pathol., Suppl. 41: 95–109, 1980. (Kato et al., 1980a.)

When the needle is inserted through the fiberoptic bronchoscope, it is kept in a retracted position to prevent damage to the instrumentation channel of the bronchoscope (Fig. 32a). A disposable syringe is attached to the needle catheter control unit, which is 95 mm long and made of stainless steel. The angle of the bevel of the needle tip is set at 15° to facilitate penetration of the bronchial wall.

Preparation for aspiration cytology is identical to that for routine fiberoptic bronchoscopy, and the procedure is performed in either the bronchoscopy room or the X-ray fluorography room.

The procedure is illustrated in Figure 34. The puncture site is first confirmed using the fiberoptic bronchoscope (1). The needle is then fully retracted and maintained in that position as it is inserted through the instrumentation channel of the fiberoptic bronchoscope to the target site, and a 20-ml disposable syringe is attached to the control unit (2). The puncture needle is then extended from its sheath (3) and advanced to perforate the wall (4). Next, aspiration is performed, and after confirming that neither air nor blood is being aspirated, the tip is moved slightly back and forth while aspirating (5). The plunger is then returned to a neutral position (6), and the needle is removed from the bronchial wall, then from the bronchoscope (7). The cells in the tip of the aspiration needle are smeared on glass slides and rapidly fixed as previously described.

The quantity of material obtained by use of the larger needle is about the same as that obtained by use of the smaller needle; but more material is obtained by the needle with the additional lateral opening. The material aspirated into the lateral orifice is cut off by the sharpened edge of the orifice as the needle is moved slightly back and forth.

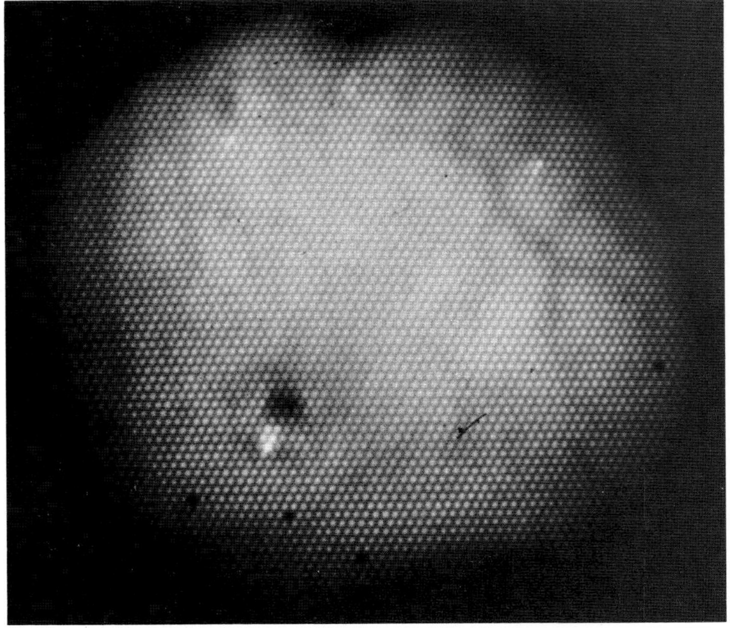

Fig. 35 The endoscopic findings after TBAC show no bleeding at the puncture site.

Complications

No complications were observed in 45 cases in which this method was performed over a 5-year period (Kato et al., 1980a), but the possibility of bleeding due to puncture of a blood vessel must be kept in mind. During pneumonectomy procedures, the authors evaluated the effects of puncture of the pulmonary artery with the 0.8-mm diameter needle. A slight degree of localized bleeding at the site of puncture of the vascular adventitial coat was recognized, but the bleeding did not last long enough to be considered serious. However, many cases of lung cancer occur in elderly patients with fragile vascular walls, in whom great care is necessary for this procedure. In addition, the operator must have a thorough knowledge of the anatomy of the lung and the distribution of the pulmonary vessels to avoid the possibility of puncture. Areas that usually do not bleed on puncture are shown in Figure 35.

Since anomalous or abnormal branching of vessels is occasionally encountered, it is advisable to evaluate the distribution of the pulmonary vessels before starting the procedure. For this purpose frontal, lateral and oblique tomograms, in addition to pulmonary and bronchial arteriograms, can be helpful.

LESION SITE AND SELECTION OF COLLECTION METHOD

The Department of Surgery of Tokyo Medical College has treated approximately 1,900 patients with lung cancer over the past 30 years, and the rates of diagnostic accuracy (Table 4) were 64.5% for sputum cytology, 81.1% for brushing/curettage cytology, 88.9% for percutaneous needle cytology and 84.2% for transbronchial aspiration cytology (TBAC), for an overall diagnostic yield of 95.8%. The rate of accuracy for each diagnostic method varied according to site (Table 5). In central type lung cancers, the rates of diagnostic accuracy were 77.7% for sputum cytology, 89.6% for brushing/curettage cytology, 83.3% for TBAC, for an overall diagnostic yield of 97.8%. In peripheral type lung cancers, the rates of diagnostic accuracy were 47.3% for sputum cytology, 70.9% for brushing/curettage cytology, 88.9% for percutaneous needle cytology and

Table 4 Lung Cancer Diagnostic Rate

Examination Methods	No. of cases	No. of positive cases	Diagnostic rate
January 1973 — August 1980 (614 cases)			
Cytological methods			
Sputum cytology	507	327	64.49%
Brushing cytology	508	412	81.10%
Percutaneous needle cytology	117	104	88.88%
TBAC*	19	16	84.21%
Histological method			
Bronchoscopic biopsy	349	285	81.66%
Preoperative or pretherapeutic diagnosis	614	588	95.76%

* Transbronchial aspiration cytology

Table 5 Diagnostic Rate according to Examination Method and Lesion of Lung Cancer

January 1973 — August 1980 (614 cases)

Examination Methods	Central type (317 cases)		Peripheral type (297 cases)	
Cytological methods				
Sputum cytology	223/287	77.70%	104/220	47.27%
Brushing cytology	249/278	89.56%	163/230	70.86%
Percutaneous needle cytology	0/0		104/117	88.88%
TBAC*	10/12	83.33%	6/7	85.71%
Histological method				
Bronchoscopic biopsy	168/186	90.32%	117/163	71.77%
Preoperative or pretherapeutic diagnosis	310/317	97.79%	278/297	93.60%

*   Transbronchial aspiration cytology

Table 6 Recent Diagnostic Rate according to Examination Method and Location

May 1978 — August 1980 (204 cases)

Examination Methods	Central type (105 cases)		Peripheral type (99 cases**)	
Cytological methods				
Sputum cytology	75/95	78.94%	42/85	50.60%
Brushing cytology	91/98	92.85%	62/77	80.51%
Percutaneous needle cytology	0/0		35/39	89.74%
TBAC*	10/12	83.33%	6/7	85.71%
Histological method				
Bronchoscopic biopsy	79/86	91.86%	42/67	61.57%
Preoperative or pretherapeutic diagnosis	105/105	100%	98/99	98.98%

*   Transbronchial aspiration cytology
** Includes four cases of positive pleural effusion.

Table 7 Diagnostic Rate according to Examination Method and Lesion Size in Peripheral Cases

January 1973 — August 1980 (297 cases)

Examination Methods	Less than 2cm (36 cases)		2 cm or more (261 cases)	
Cytological methods				
Sputum cytology	8/31	25.80%	96/187	51.33%
Brushing cytology	19/31	61.29%	144/199	72.36%
Percutaneous needle cytology	18/21	85.71%	86/96	89.58%
TBAC*	1/1	100%	5/6	83.33%
Histological methods				
Bronchoscopic biopsy	4/9	44.44%	110/150	73.33%

*   Transbronchial aspiration cytology

85.7% for TBAC for an overall diagnostic accuracy of 93.6%. These rates are for the 8-year period of 1973—1980, in which a total of 614 cases were examined, but developments in diagnostic procedures and technique have since yielded a 100% diagnostic accuracy in central type lung cancers and an accuracy of 98.9% for peripheral type cancers (Table 6).

Table 7 shows the diagnostic yield of peripheral type lung cancers according to size. The diagnostic accuracies for lesions less than 2 cm in greatest dimension were 25.8% for sputum cytology, 61.3% for brushing/curettage cytology, 85.7% for percutaneous needle cytology and 100% for TBAC. The diagnostic yields for lesions more than 2 cm in greatest dimension were 51.3% for sputum cytology, 72.4% for brushing/curettage cytology, 89.6% for percutaneous needle cytology and 83.3% for TBAC (Kato et al., 1981c).

These data indicate that in central type lung cancers, the most effective cytologic diagnostic method is transfiberoptic bronchoscopic brushing/curettage cytology. Sputum cytologic diagnosis is also effective in the diagnosis of central type lung cancer and it has special importance in the diagnosis of early stage central type lung cancer cases, which frequently do not exhibit abnormalities on chest X-ray films. TBAC is effective in cases in which the lesion is covered by normal epithelium, although the number of such cases is small (Figs. 36—38).

In peripheral type lung cancers, percutaneous needle cytology is the most effective method, and its diagnostic yield is almost unrelated to the size of the lesion. In cases of peripheral type lung cancers in which the lesions are larger than 2 cm in greatest dimension, brushing/curettage cytology performed under X-ray

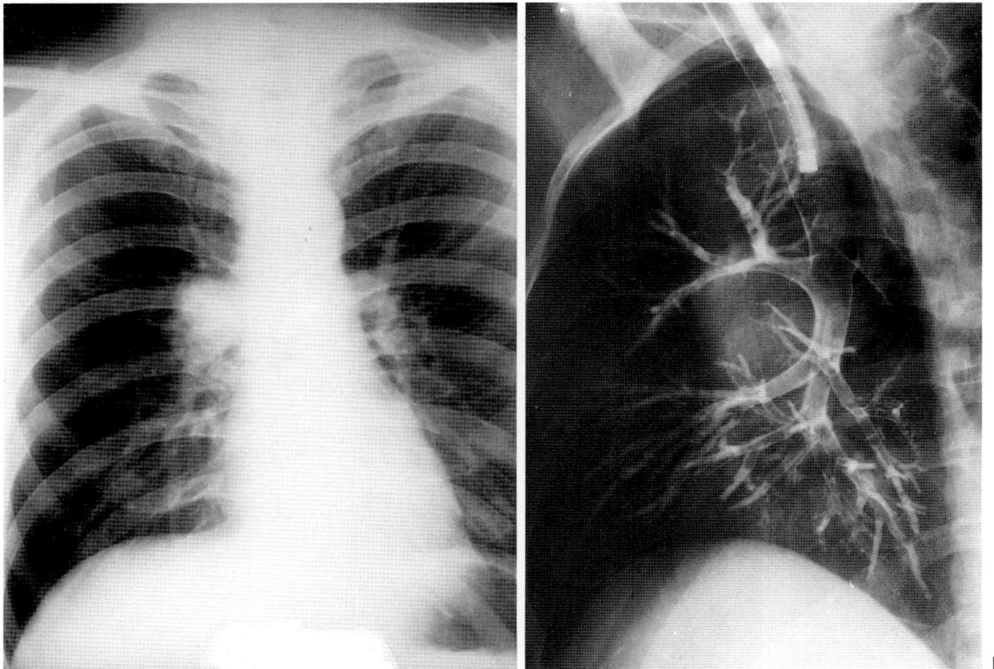

Fig. 36 This case showed widening of the bifurcation between the right upper lobe bronchus and the truncus intermedius. (a) Chest X-ray film. (b) Bronchogram.

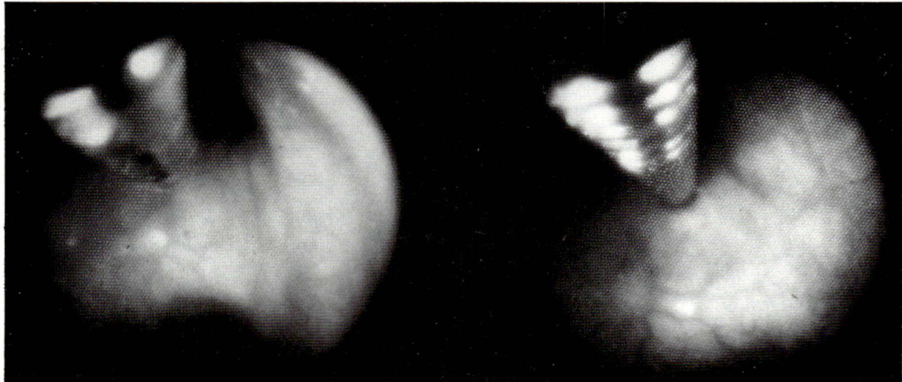

Fig. 37 TBAC procedure in the case shown in Figure 36. The needle is inserted into the bifurcation of the right upper lobe bronchus and the truncus intermedius. No mucosal abnormalities were recognized. TBAC revealed carcinoid.
Previously published in Hayata, Y. (ed.): Lung Cancer Diagnosis, Igaku-Shoin, Tokyo and New York, 1982. (From Kato, H. and Ono, J., 1982.)

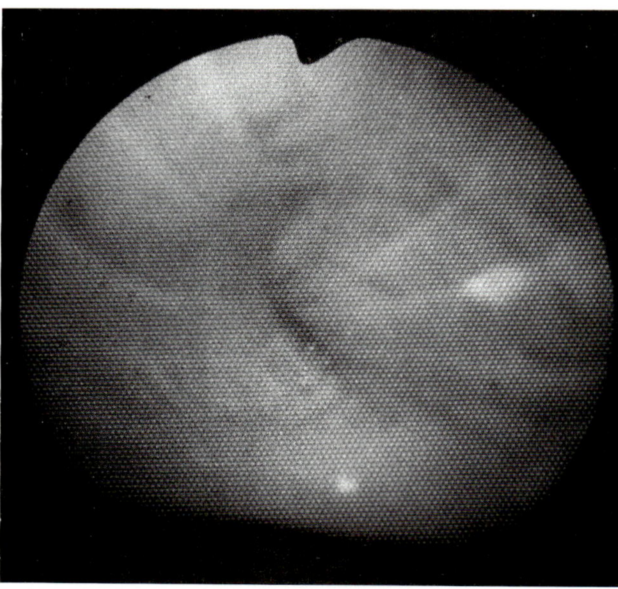

Fig. 38 Obstruction of the right upper lobe bronchus was recognized but biopsy and brushing obtained no diagnostic material. However TBAC, obtaining material beyond the mucosa, yielded a diagnosis of small cell carcinoma.

television guidance is also an effective method. Sputum cytology is ineffective in cases of peripheral lesions less than 2 cm in greatest dimension (Table 8).

Table 9 shows the rate of diagnostic accuracy in relation to histologic type and diagnostic method. Since the majority of squamous cell carcinomas develop as a central type lung lesion, sputum cytology, brushing/curettage cytology and TBAC are all effective diagnostic methods. On the other hand, since adenocarcinoma tends to originate peripherally, the highest diagnostic yields are obtained using percutaneous needle cytology, TBAC (Fig. 39) and brushing/currettage cytology. In small cell carcinoma, which occurs less frequently, the diagnostic yields were 100% for percutaneous needle cytology and 64% for sputum cytology. In large cell carcinoma, the number of percutaneous needle cytology and TBAC cases was

Table 8 Indications of collection methods according to the lesion characteristics

	Sputum cytology	Bronchoscopic brushing & curettage cytology	Transbronchial needle aspiration cytology	Percutaneous needle cytology
Central type				
Superficial growth	Indicated	Indicated	Not indicated	Not indicated
Submucosal growth	Not indicated	Not indicated	Indicated	Not indicated
Periperal type				
More than 2cm	Indicated	Indicated	Indicated	Indicated
Less than 2cm	Not indicated	Indicated	Indicated	Indicated

low, therefore the diagnostic accuracies were not evaluated, but the yields for brushing/currettage cytology and sputum cytology were 90.9% and 72.7%, respectively.

Cytologic harvesting of specimens via the fiberoptic bronchoscope yielded the highest diagnostic rate, but it is important to remember that squamous cell carcinoma is often accompanied by necrosis. Therefore, when collecting specimens, it is necessary to penetrate beyond the necrotic portion.

Table 9 Diagnostic Accuracy according to Histological Type and Examination Method

May 1978 — August 1980 (204 cases)

Histological Types & Examination Method	sq. cell ca. (59 cases)	adeno ca. (99 cases)	small cell ca. (30 cases)	large cell ca. (13 cases)	mucoepi. ca. adenoid cyst. ca., carcino-sarcoma (3 cases)	
Cytological methods						
Sputum cytology	47/59 79.66%	45/79 56.96%	16/25 64.0%	8/11 72.72%	0/3	0%
Brushing cytology	49/52 94.23%	61/77 79.22%	24/29 82.75%	10/11 90.90%	3/3	100%
Percutaneous needle cytology	9/11 81.81%	18/19 94.73%	8/8 100%	2/2 100%	0/0	
TBAC*	4/4 100%	5/6 83.33%	2/4 50%	3/3 100%	1/1	100%
Histological method						
Bronchoscopic biopsy	37/43 86.01%	54/74 72.97%	16/19 84.21%	11/12 91.66%	2/3	66.66%

* Transbronchial aspiration cytology

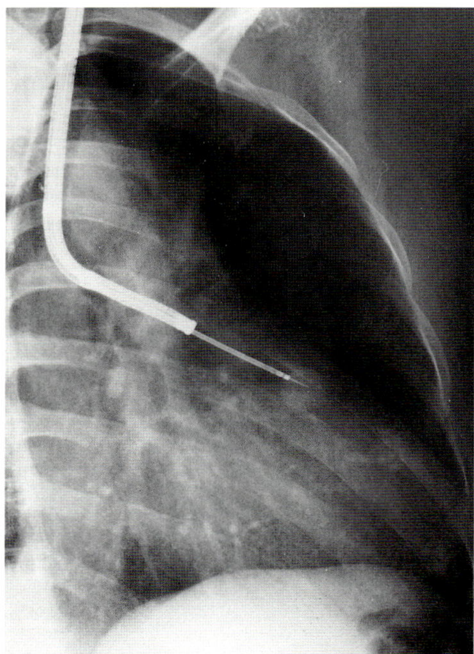

Fig. 39 TBAC in a peripheral lesion case. This method is indicated for lesions from which materials cannot be harvested by conventional bronchoscopic techniques.

II

Basic Structure of
the Respiratory Tract

UPPER RESPIRATORY TRACT

The upper respiratory tract consists of the nasal cavity, oral cavity, pharynx and
larynx. Material from the epithelium of all these regions can appear in sputum
cytology specimens.

Most of the nasal cavity is covered by squamous epithelium and ciliated columnar epithelium intermingled with occasional goblet cells can also be seen in parts.
The oral cavity is linked with stratified squamous epithelium, as is the mesopharynx and hypopharynx. However the upper pharynx is lined with ciliated columnar cell. The larynx is covered by a combination of ciliated columnar cells and
stratified squamous epithelium (Fig. 40).

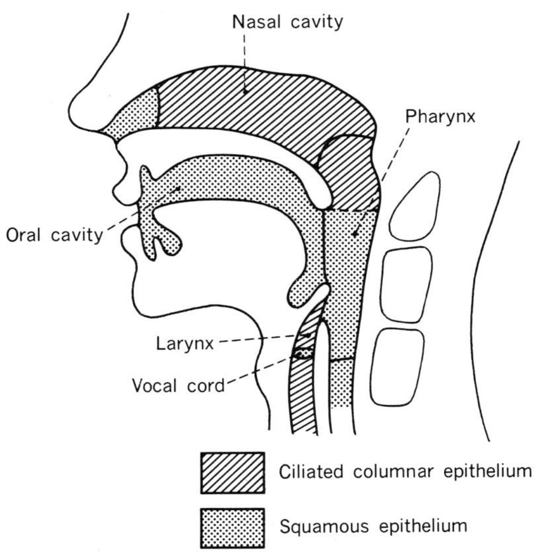

Fig. 40 Cytological distribution in the upper respiratory tract.

LOWER RESPIRATORY TRACT

The lower respiratory tract consists of the trachea, bronchi and alveoli. The trachea bifurcates to the left and right main bronchi which then branch to successively smaller bronchi, bronchioles, terminal bronchioles, respiratory bronchioles, alveolar ducts and alveoli (Fig. 41).

Most of the trachea and bronchi are lined with ciliated columnar cells (Fig. 42) intermittently sprinkled with goblet cells at a ratio of 5:1 to 6:1 (Rhodin, 1966). The basal portion usually is composed of basal cells above which are located the intermediate cells that are thought to differentiate to goblet cells and to ciliated columnar cells. However it is difficult to distinguish between intermediate cells and basal cells on the basis of conventional light microscopy.

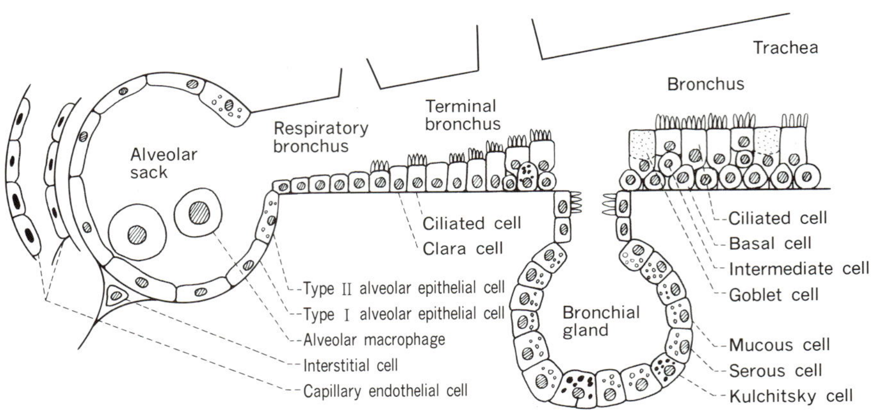

Fig. 41 Cytological distribution from the trachea to alveolus. (Lining of mucous, serous and Kulchitsky cells)

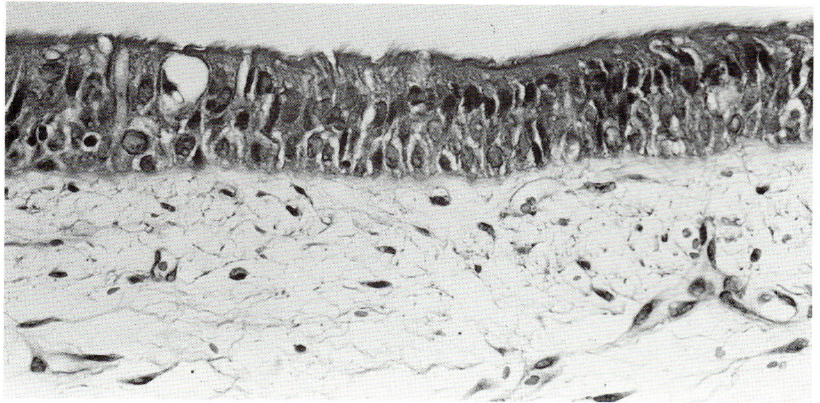

Fig. 42 Histologic findings of the normal bronchus. The major bronchial structure consists of ciliated columnar cells, goblet cells, intermediate cells and basal cells. (×100, H.E.*) (* Hematoxylin-eosion stain)

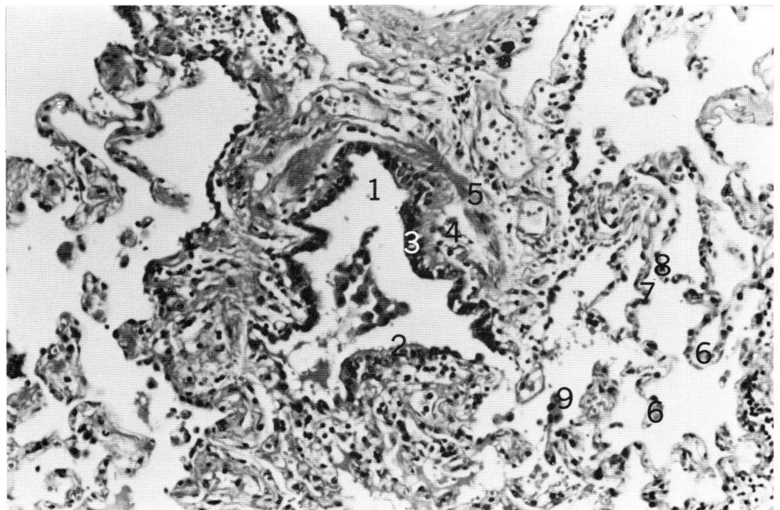

Fig. 43 Bronchiole and alveoli. The bronchiolar epithelium is composed of low columnar ciliated cells, cuboidal cells, thin lamina propria and smooth muscle. Mucosal folds are remarkable.(x40, H.E.)

1. Bronchiole
2. Low ciliated columnar cells
3. Cuboidal cells
4. Lamina propia
5. Smooth muscle fiber
6. Capillary
7. Intraalveolar-septal connective tissue
8. Alveolar cells
9. Alveolar macrophages

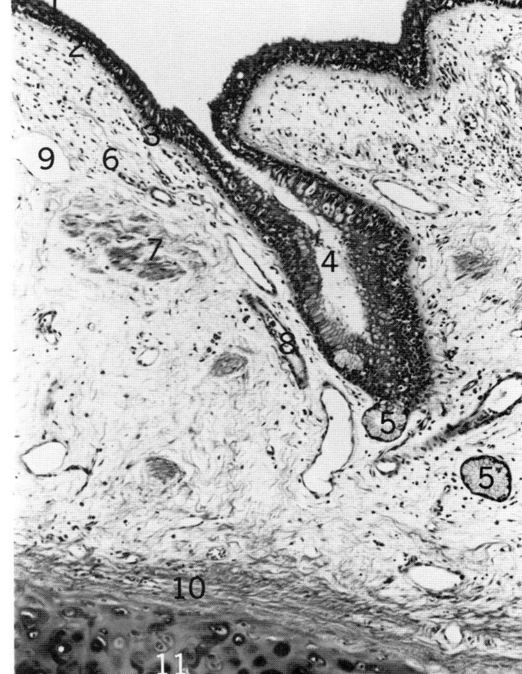

Fig. 44 Bronchial gland consists of duct and alveoli. The alveoli consist of mucous and serous alveoli. (x40, H.E.)

1. Ciliated columnar cells
2. Basal cells
3. Basement membrane
4. Duct of bronchial gland
5. Bronchial glands
6. Lamina propria
7. Smooth muscle fibers
8. Vessels
9. Lymph duct
10. Perichondrium
11. Cartilage

Goblet cells appear less frequently in segmental bronchi and disappear completely in bronchioles. Basal cells disappear distal from terminal bronchioles. Basal cells can only be seen up to, but not including terminal bronchioles. In terminal bronchioles and more distal areas only ciliated columnar cells (Clara cells) can be recognized (Fig. 43). These cells gradually become increasingly cuboidal with cilia disappearing as the transition to alveoli occurs.

Alveoli are made up of alveolar epithelial cells, alveolar macrophages, interstitial cells and capillary endothelial cells (see Fig. 43). There are two types of alveolar epithelial cells, type I alveolar epithelial cells which are small epithelial alveolar cells and type II alveolar epithelial cells which are alveolar wall cells containing osmiophilic lamellar bodies in the cytoplasm. However it is impossible to distinguish between these two types by light microscopy (Spencer, 1977; Takahashi, 1981).

Lying in the bronchial submucosal layer are bronchial glands (Fig. 44) consisting of two types of secretory cells, mucous cells and serous cells and Kulchitsky cells (Bensch et al., 1965).

III

Normal Respiratory Cells

SPUTUM SPECIMENS

Normal epithelial cells that are observed in sputum specimens include squamous epithelial cells, ciliated columnar cells, goblet cells and basal cells. In addition, nonepithelial cells, such as alveolar macrophages, lymphocytes (Fig. 45) and neutrophils (Fig. 46) are recognized in sputum specimens even from healthy persons.

Most squamous epithelial cells observed in sputum derive from the oral cavity, mesopharynx and hypopharynx. Many superficial cells show keratinization, with a wide range of morphologic findings. Cytoplasm is thin, with occasional superimposition or convergence. Stainability indicates eosinophilic characteristics. Granular keratohyalin can sometimes be recognized in the cytoplasm. Nuclei are small and rounded. The nuclear to cytoplasmic (N/C) ratio is very low (Fig. 47). Cells of the deep layer of the squamous epithelium are almost round, and they are smaller than cells of the superficial epithelium and have slightly larger nuclei. The

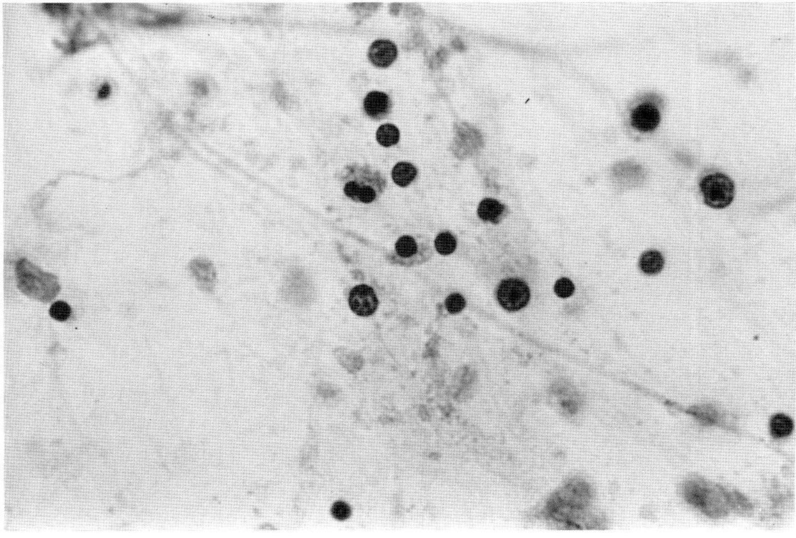

Fig. 45 Lymphocytes in sputum. Round and small (4—5 μ in size) cells with scanty cytoplasm are observed. (X400, Pap.)

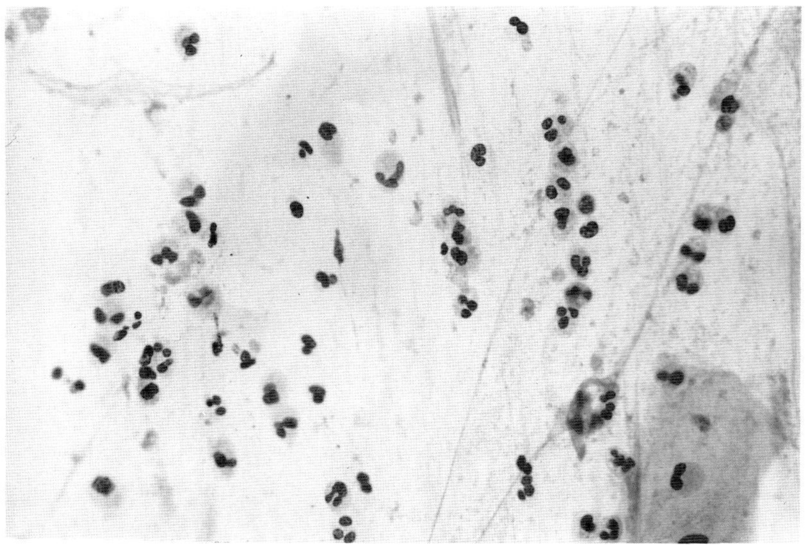

Fig. 46 Leucocytes in sputum. Segmented nuclei staining basophilically are characteristic. This specimen was obtained from a patient with pneumonia. (X400, Pap.)

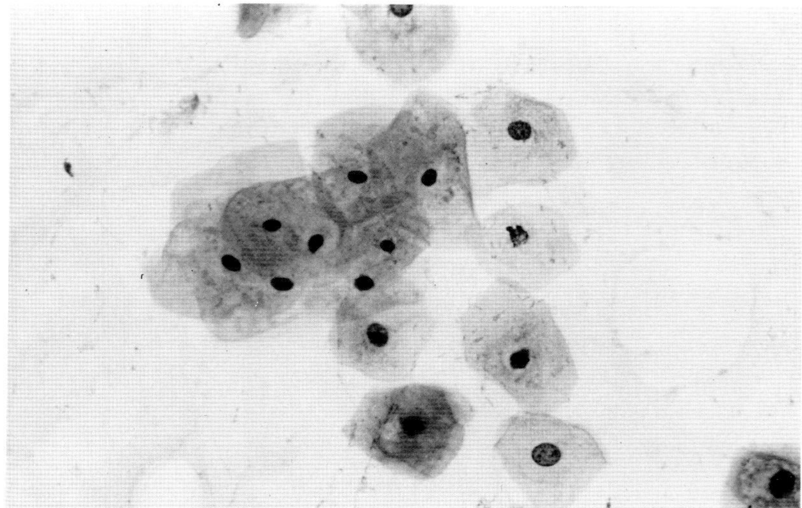

Fig. 47 Oral squamous cells in sputum. These cells were obtained from the surface layer of the squamous epithelium of the oral cavity and pharynx. N/C ratio is very small. (X400, Pap.)

cytoplasm shows a basophilic staining pattern. The N/C ratio is higher (Fig. 48). At times, groups of these cells are important in making a differential diagnosis of squamous metaplasia.

Degenerated ciliated columnar epithelial cells appear with poor stainability in routine sputum specimens but are also often seen in sputum expectorated after fiberoptic bronchoscopy. They are morphologically either columnar or spindle shaped, with a tail on one side. The side with cilia is referred to as the terminal plate and is slightly reddish yellow on Papanicolaou stain. The nucleus is closer to

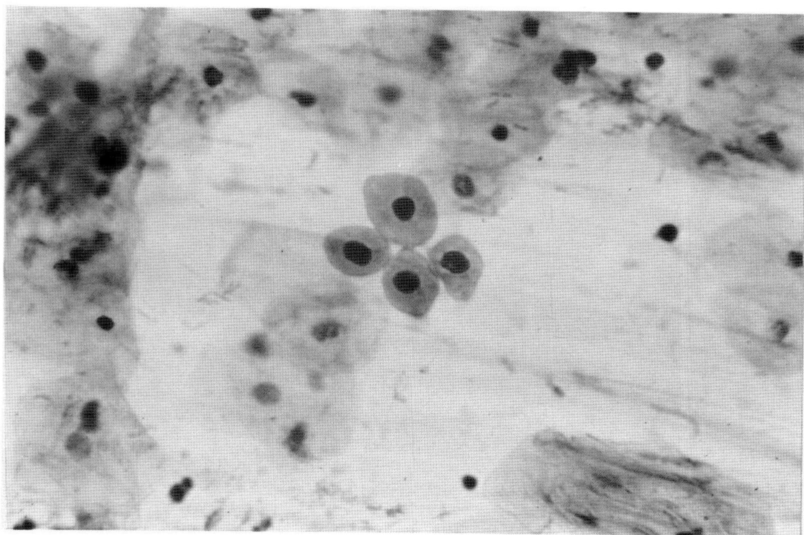

Fig. 48 Oral squamous cells in sputum. These smaller cells derived from the deep layer of the squamous epithelium. (X400, Pap.)

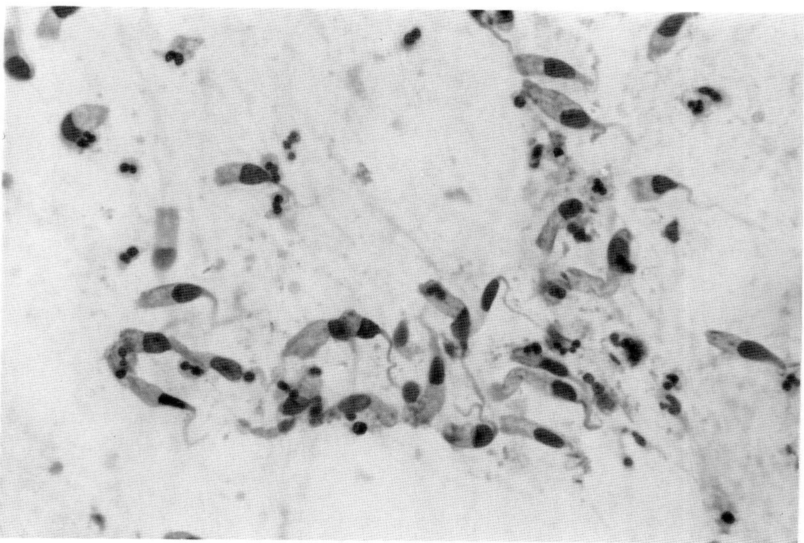

Fig. 49 Columnar cells in sputum. These exfoliated columnar cells in sputum show cellular degeneration. (X400, Pap.)

the tail, rounded and possesses fine granular chromatin. Some cells have one or two nucleoli. Cilia detach easily, therefore in most columnar cells in sputum the cilia have detached leaving only the terminal plate (Fig. 49).

Goblet cells are infrequently encountered in sputum specimens from healthy persons. The cytoplasm possesses large vacuoles, and the nucleus is located eccentrically toward the tail. The nucleus is occasionally deformed by secretory vacuoles (Fig. 50).

Basal cells are almost circular, with relatively large, round nuclei possessing fine granular chromatin. A small nucleolus can sometimes be recognized (Fig. 51). Basal cells are rarely seen in sputum specimens from healthy persons, and if they appear in clusters, the possibility of basal cell hyperplasia must be considered. Basal cells must be distinguished from small cell carcinoma, carcinoid and lymphocytes.

In sputum specimens, the presence of nonepithelial alveolar macrophages is an extremely important finding. The presence of such macrophages indicates that the sputum derives from the deeper portion of the respiratory tract, whereas their

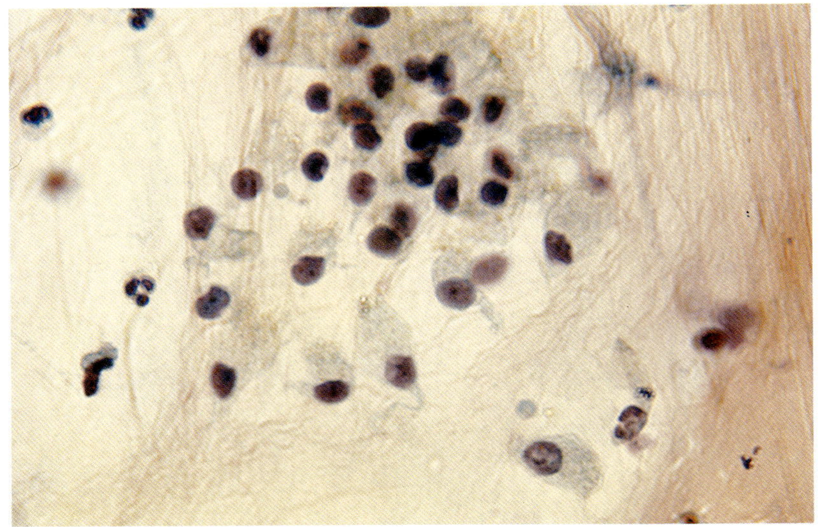

Fig. 50 Goblet cells in sputum. Cytoplasmic vacuolization is observed. The cells show degeneration in sputum. This specimen was obtained from a patient with chronic bronchitis. (X400, Pap.)

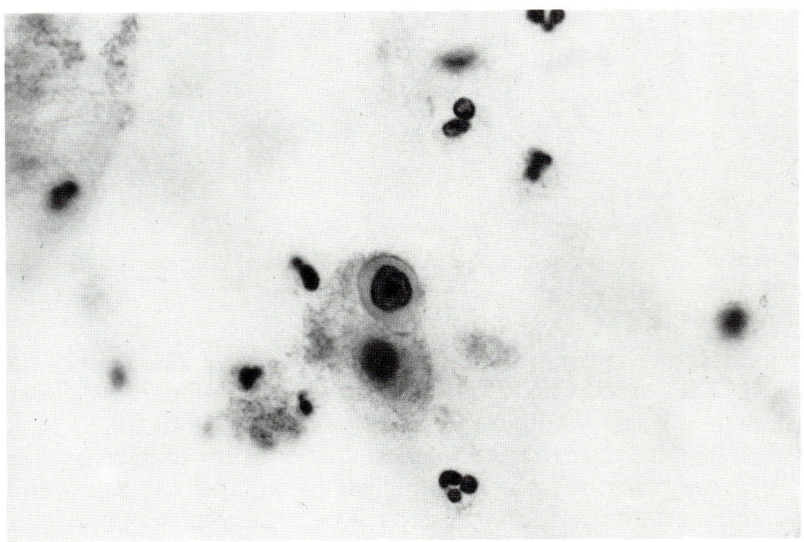

Fig. 51 Basal cells in sputum. A round nucleus and large N/C ratio are characteristic. (X400, Pap.)

absence indicates that the specimen is not satisfactory. Alveolar macrophages are generally round, and their cytoplasm contains small vacuoles. They are frequently observed to have engulfed macroscopic foreign bodies, such as anthracotic particles (Fig. 52). The nuclei are either round, oval or kidney-shaped, located eccentrically and partially in contact with the cytoplasm. The chromatin is granular, and the nuclear membrane can be clearly recognized. One or two nucleoli can sometimes be distinguished, and multinucleated cells are occasionally seen (Fig. 53).

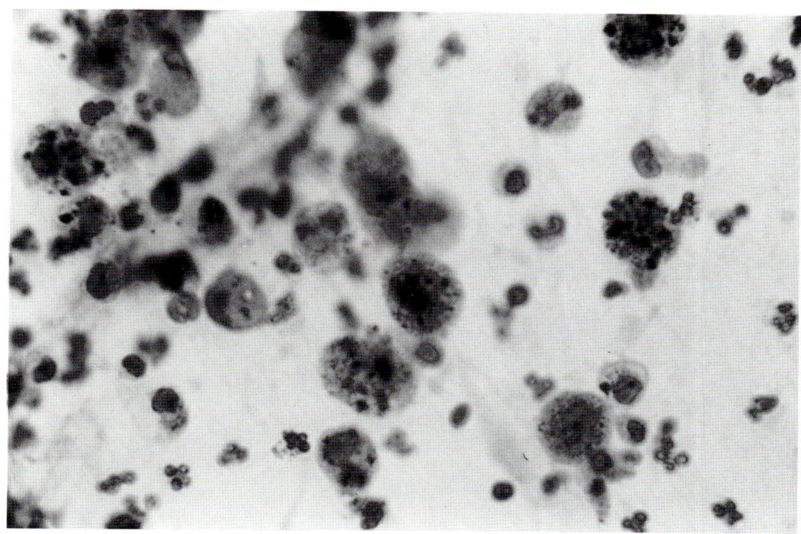

Fig. 52 Alveolar macrophages in sputum. Much foreign material is observed in their cytoplasm. This specimen was obtained from a heavy smoker. (X400, Pap.)

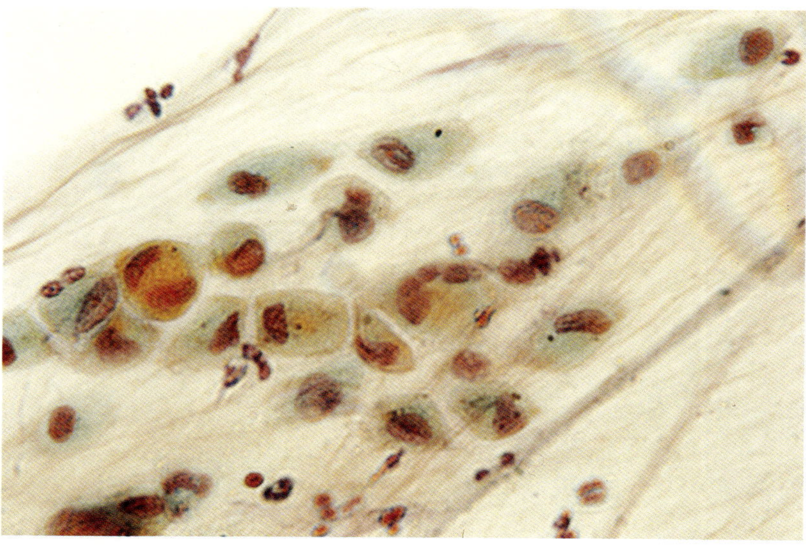

Fig. 53 Alveolar macrophages in sputum. The nucleus is kidney-shaped or folded with foamy cytoplasm. Some cells have two nuclei. (X400, Pap.)

FIBEROPTIC BRONCHOSCOPIC BRUSHING SPECIMENS

Normal epithelial cells observed in materials obtained by fiberoptic bronchoscopic brushing include ciliated columnar epithelial cells, goblet cells and basal cells.

Most cells are usually ciliated columnar epithelial cells (Fig. 54), which often

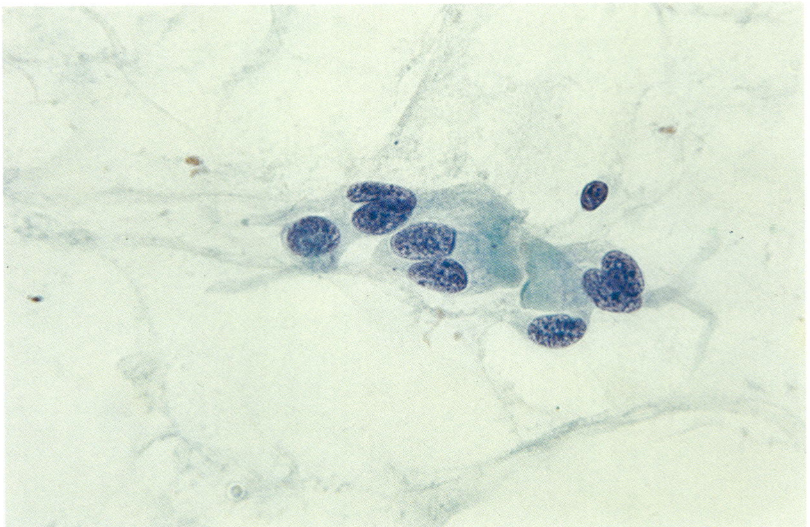

Fig. 54 Columnar cells in a brushing specimen. Cilia are well preserved in this brushing specimen showing little degeneration. (X400, Pap.)

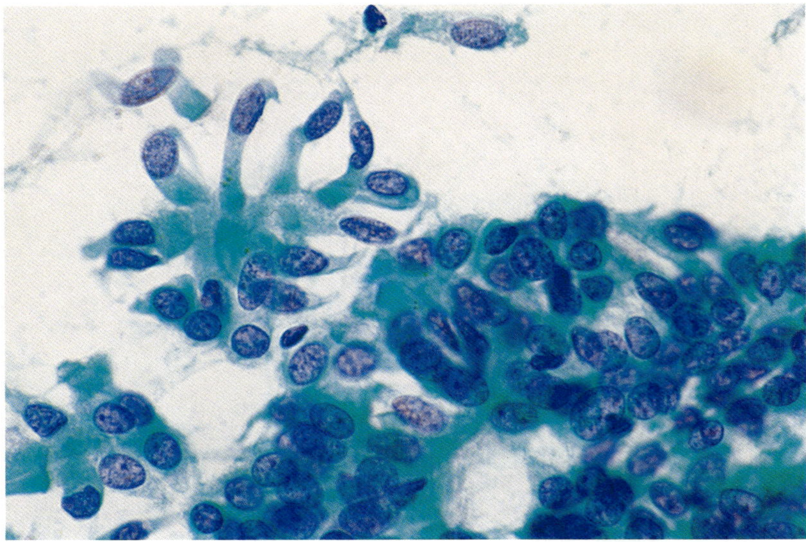

Fig. 55 Columnar cells in a brushing specimen. Occasionally cells were obtained in clusters. This is characteristic of brushing specimens. (X400, Pap.)

appear in clusters due to the mechanical method of harvesting. Large clusters appear occasionally (Fig. 55). Normal cells obtained by transbronchial brushing show little morphologic degeneration, and cilia are well preserved.

Goblet cells usually appear intermingled with ciliated columnar epithelial cells. In brushing materials, the cytologic degeneration is minimal; therefore, mucus in the cytoplasm stains pink or brown and the nucleoli are well preserved (Fig. 56). The basal cells are easily observed in the specimen. The cells are small but larger than lymphocytes. The cytoplasm is scanty, and because of the relatively large

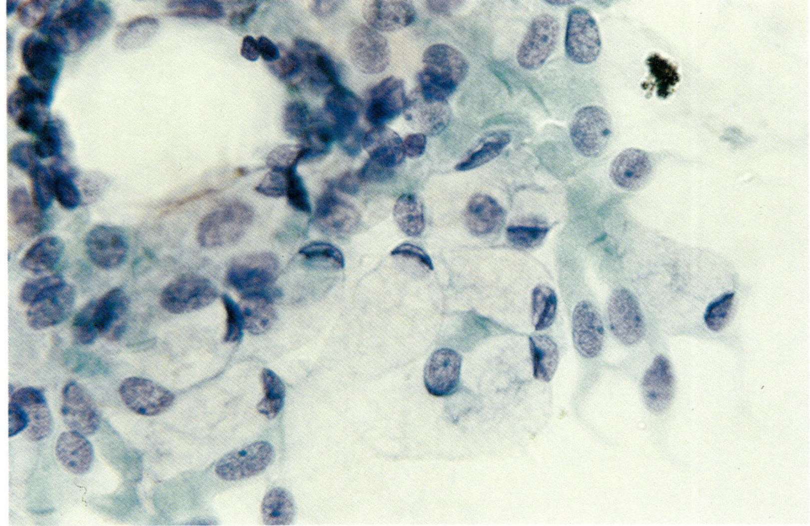

Fig. 56 Well preserved goblet cells in a brushing specimen containing mucus. (X400, Pap.)

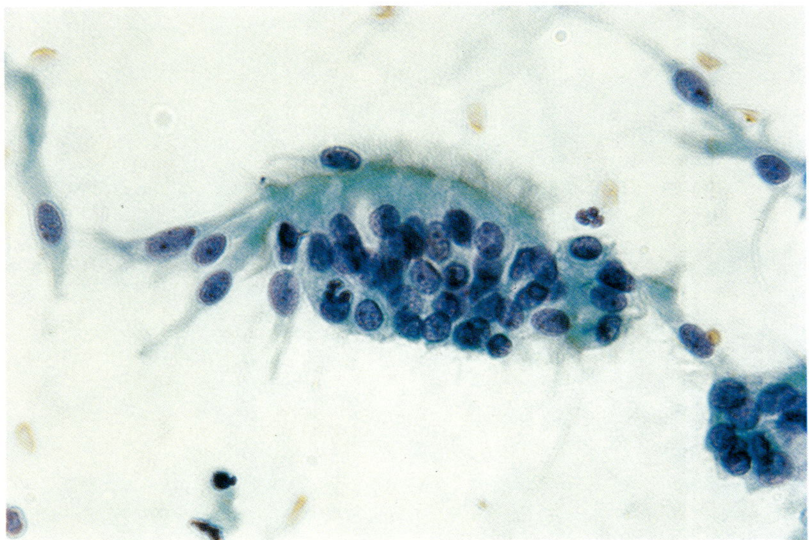

Fig. 57 Basal and columnar cells in a brushing specimen. Brushing enables collection of cells from the entire epithelial layer of the bronchial wall. Basal cells can be seen under the columnar cells. They are small round cells with a large N/C ratio. (X400, Pap.)

nuclei, there is a high N/C ratio. The nuclei are round and have fine granular chromatin showing no degeneration. These cells are frequently observed to adhere to the ciliated columnar cells (Fig. 57).

Specimens obtained by brushing under X-ray television guidance can include low ciliated columnar cells and cuboidal cells from the terminal bronchi.

BRONCHIAL LAVAGE SPECIMENS

Most of the cells obtained by this technique are columnar cells (Fig. 58), basal cells, bronchioloalveolar cells and macrophages. With this method, since cellular degeneration occurs easily, it is necessary to give careful consideration to the fixation technique. We use a container of 5 ml of 50% alcohol solution as the fixative.

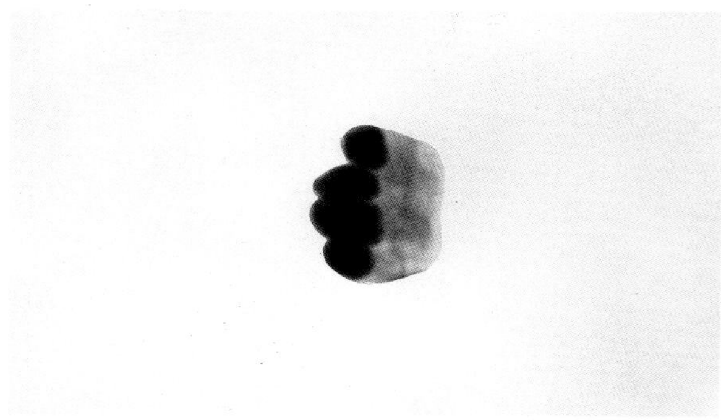

Fig. 58 Low ciliated columnar cells from peripheral bronchi in a bronchial lavage specimen. (X400, Pap.)

NEEDLE CYTOLOGY SPECIMENS

Normal cells obtained by needle puncture include ciliated columnar epithelial cells, bronchioloalveolar epithelial cells, alveolar interstitial connective tissue cells, alveolar macrophages and blood components.

Most ciliated epithelial cells obtained from the terminal bronchi are relatively low, and small. Cuboidal cells are also occasionally recognized.

Terminal bronchiolar cells or hyperplastic type 2 alveolar cells are relatively small and round or cuboidal, and many small vacuoles can be observed in their cytoplasm. The nuclei are small and round and have granular chromatin (Fig. 59). Alveolar epithelial cells are sometimes mistaken for alveolar macrophages (Johnston and Frable, 1976).

Interstitial connective tissue cells are often seen in specimens obtained by means of a fine needle with protrusions (Fig. 60).

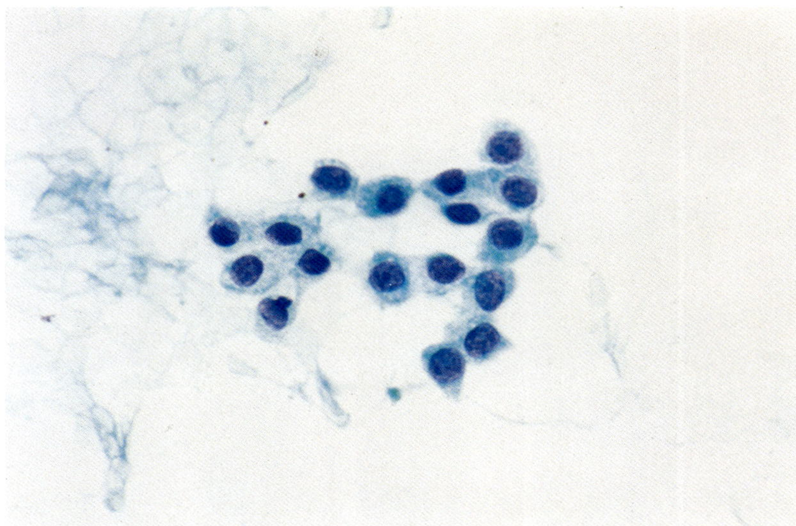

Fig. 59 Bronchioloalveolar cells in needle cytology specimen. Small, round or cuboidal cells with fine granular chromatins are characteristic. (X400, Pap.)

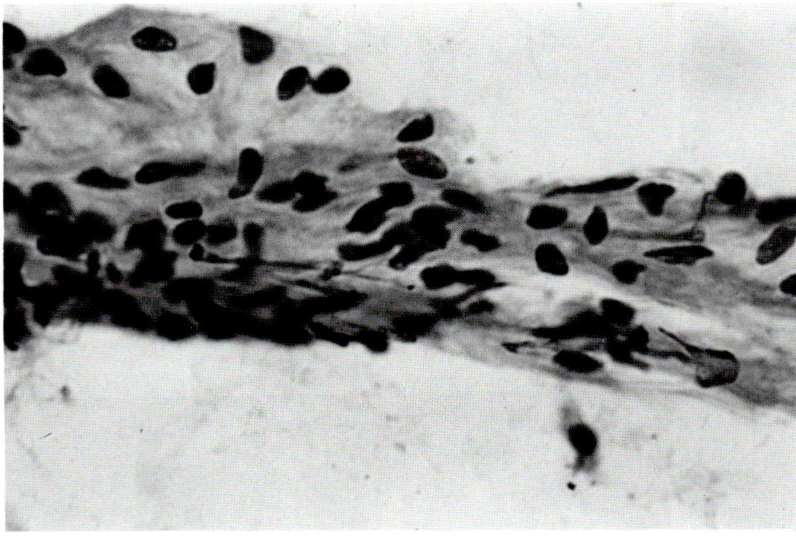

Fig. 60 Interstitial connective tissue cells in a needle cytology specimen. Spindle cells with elongated nuclei are present. (X400, Pap.)

IV

Cytologic Diagnosis of Benign Findings of the Respiratory Tract

EPITHELIAL CELLS

Abnormal Columnar Cells

Ciliated columnar epithelial cells are highly responsive to stimuli and inflammation. Nuclear hypertrophy and multinucleation are often observed, as are an increase in the amount of nuclear chromatin and multiple hypertrophic nucleoli. Marked nuclear atypia is occasionally recognized, but the benign nature of the disease is revealed by the retention of cilia on the terminal plate (Fig. 61).

Ciliocytophthoria

This term is used to describe a type of degeneration of ciliated columnar epithelial cells in which the ciliated cytoplasm appears to be detached from the portion containing the degenerated nucleus (Papanicolaou, 1956; Papanicolaou et al., 1961). The cytoplasm frequently contains eosinophilic inclusions (Fig. 62).

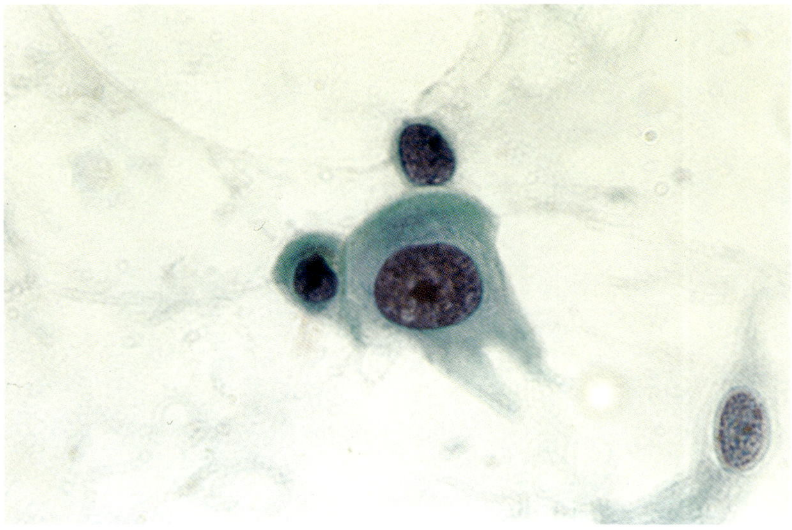

Fig. 61 Abnormal columnar cell in a brushing cytology specimen. The nucleus has increased in size with a prominent nucleolus and the chromatin is increased in quantity. A terminal plate indicates this cell still benign status (from chronic bronchitis). (X400, Pap.)

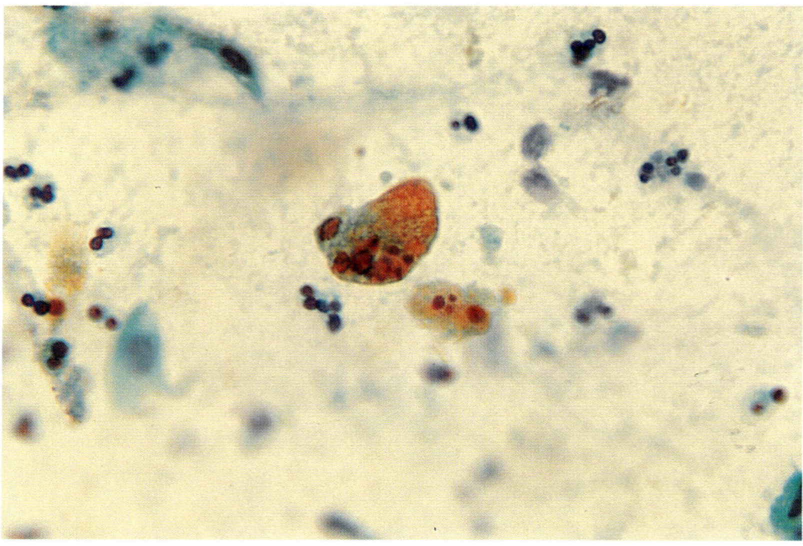

Fig. 62 Ciliocytophthoria cells in a sputum cytology specimen. Eosinophilic granules are included in the cytoplasm. The nucleus is destroyed (from chronic bronchitis). (X400, Pap.)

Ciliocytophthoria (C.C.P.) is frequently recognized in cases of viral infection, bacterial infection or malignant tumor. Therefore, the possibility of a malignant tumor must be considered in cases of C.C.P.

Inclusion bodies
Inclusion bodies are a characteristic finding in viral infections and are thought to form as a result of indentation of the cytoplasm into the nucleus (Fig. 63) (Naib et al., 1968; Coleman, 1975).

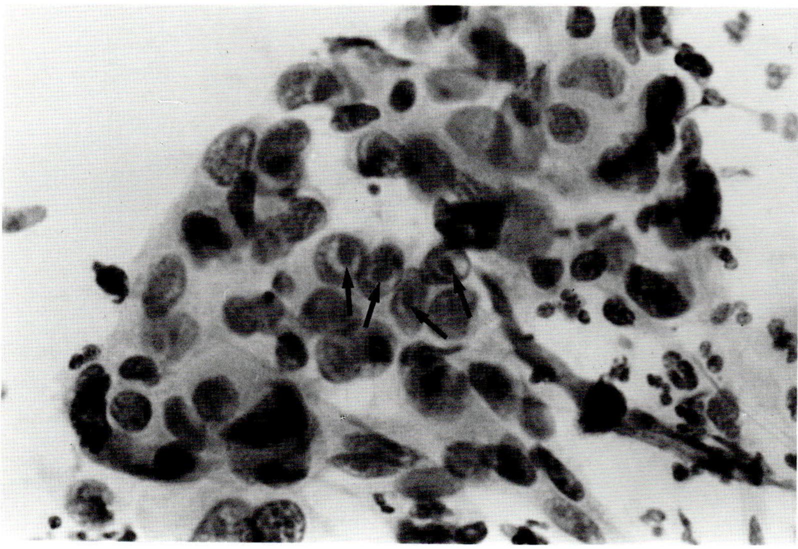

Fig. 63 Inclusion bodies are seen in the nuclei of this sputum cytology specimen from a case of cytomegaloviral infection (arrows). The inclusion bodies are larger than the nucleoli and are surrounded by haloes. (Courtesy of Dr. H. Koketsu, National Cancer Center Hospital, Tokyo) (X400, Pap.)

Columnar Epithelial Cell Hyperplasia

Since the columnar epithelial cells of the terminal bronchi can display adenomatous proliferation due to chronic bronchitis, fibrosis of the lung or airway burn, when clusters of such cells are exfoliated in sputum, they can strongly resemble adenocarcinoma (Fig. 64). Columnar cell hyperplasia seen in sputum specimens usually appears as a tightly packed arrangement of cells that takes the form of a tight, smooth-surfaced ball. Some cells have abundant cytoplasm and exhibit vacuolation. Variation in nuclear size is sometimes seen, but the chromatin pattern is uniform. Cells with hypertrophic nucleoli are sometimes observed.

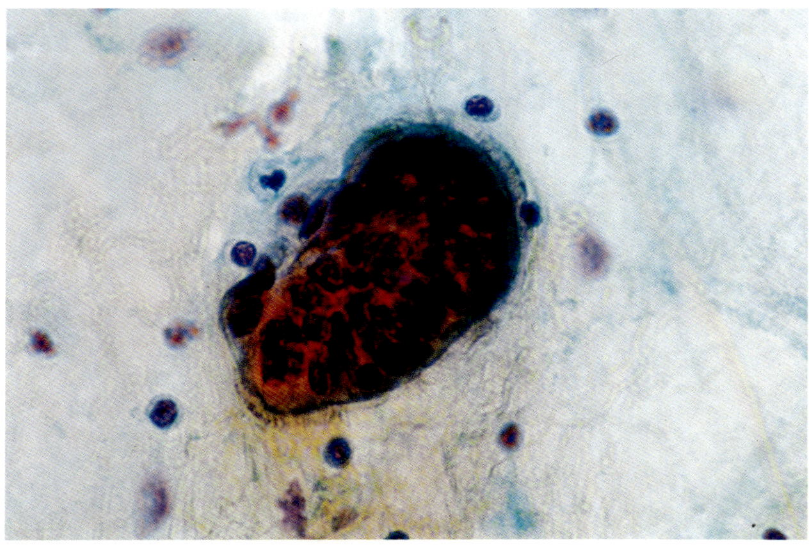

Fig. 64 Cluster of columnar cells in a sputum cytology specimen. This shows proliferation of columnar epithelial cells. Cells at the border of the tight clusters show little variation in nuclear size and homogenous chromatin pattern with cilia (from bronchial asthma). (X400, Pap.)

Columnar epithelial cell hyperplasia can be distinguished from papillary adenocarcinoma, especially bronchioloalveolar cell carcinoma, on the basis of two findings. The cilia or their shadows can be recognized and nuclear atypia is not marked in columnar epithelial cell hyperplasia in a benign condition.

Goblet Cell Hyperplasia

A variety of stimuli can easily produce goblet cell hyperplasia. This type of hyperplasia is often accompanied by basal cell hyperplasia in heavy smokers.

Hyperplasia of goblet cells results in an increase in bronchial secretions which can be thought to protect the normal bronchial mucosa from foreign bodies and other noncellular elements.

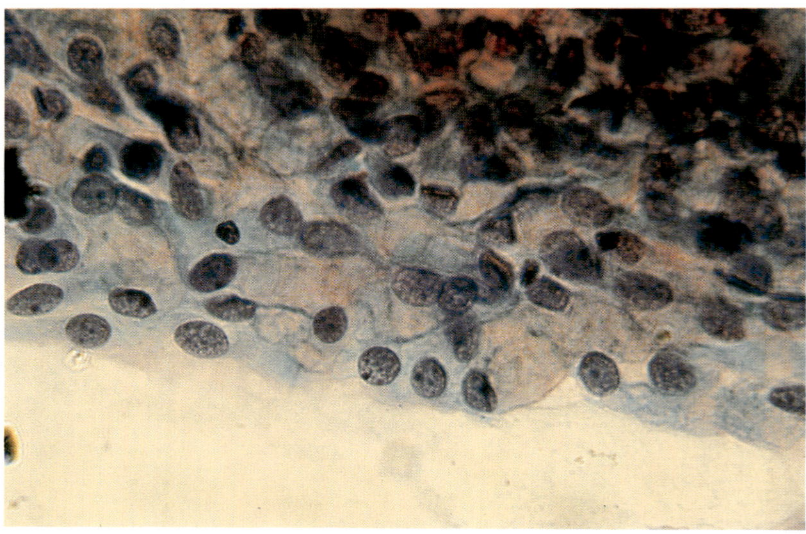

Fig. 65 Goblet cell hyperplasia in a brushing cytology specimen. The cluster consists mainly of goblet cells (from chronic bronchitis). (X400, Pap.)

A diagnosis of goblet cell hyperplasia can be made if clusters of these cells are seen in the cytology specimen. Sputum specimens show degeneration to some degree (See Fig. 56), whereas brushing specimens demonstrate less degeneration (Fig. 65).

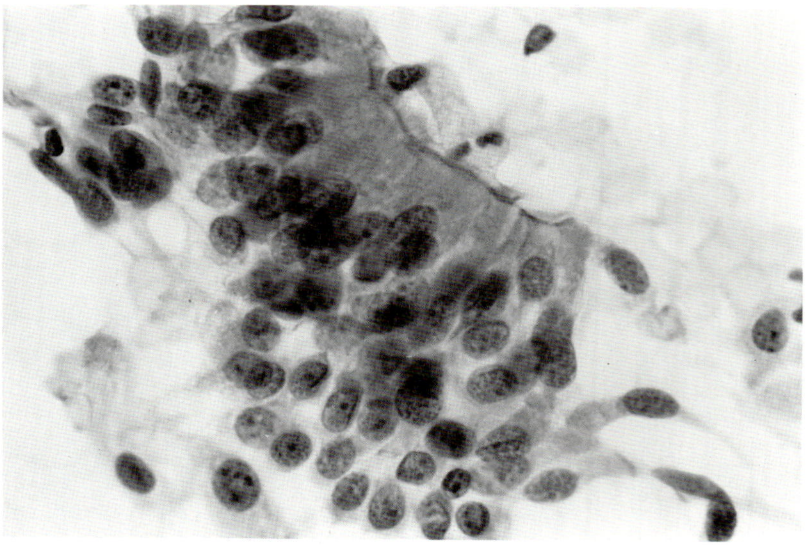

Fig. 66 Basal cell hyperplasia in a brushing cytology specimen. Most of the cluster consists of basal cells. Ciliated columnar epithelial cells can be recognized in some parts of the cluster of cells (from chronic bronchitis). (X400, Pap.)

Basal Cell Hyperplasia

Hyperplasia of basal cells, which are located in airways larger than bronchioles, can occur in response to a variety of conditions and agents, such as chronic inflammation, tobacco smoke or exposure to carcinogens. Basal cell hyperplasia is observed with or without ciliated columnar cells. Clusters of these cells are frequently observed in bronchial brushing specimens. Proliferation of basal cells is sometimes accompanied by increases in the size of nuclei and in the amount of chromatin, hypertrophic nucleoli can be seen and care must be taken to distinguish such cells from carcinoma cells. Cells appearing in clusters show good cellular adherence. The definition of basal cell hyperplasia is based on the occurrence of clusters composed of numerous basal cells (Fig. 66).

Differentiation from carcinoma cells can be made on the basis of the presence of ciliated columnar cells in some of the clusters and the relatively regular nuclear shape and the homogeneous distribution of the granular nuclear chromatin. The possibility of a relationship between basal cell hyperplasia and squamous metaplasia is currently under investigation (Ide et al., 1966; Kato et al., 1980b).

Cellular Changes Due To Therapy

Radiotherapy and chemotherapy can cause changes in bronchial epithelial cells to produce a morphologic resemblance to cancer cells (Figs. 67 and 68). When such changes occur in ciliated columnar cells, they can be diagnosed as benign on the basis of the presence of cilia or a terminal plate, but when treatment causes the basal cells to change to cells that show less differentiation than basal cells, it is difficult to distinguish them from cancer cells morphologically. The cellular

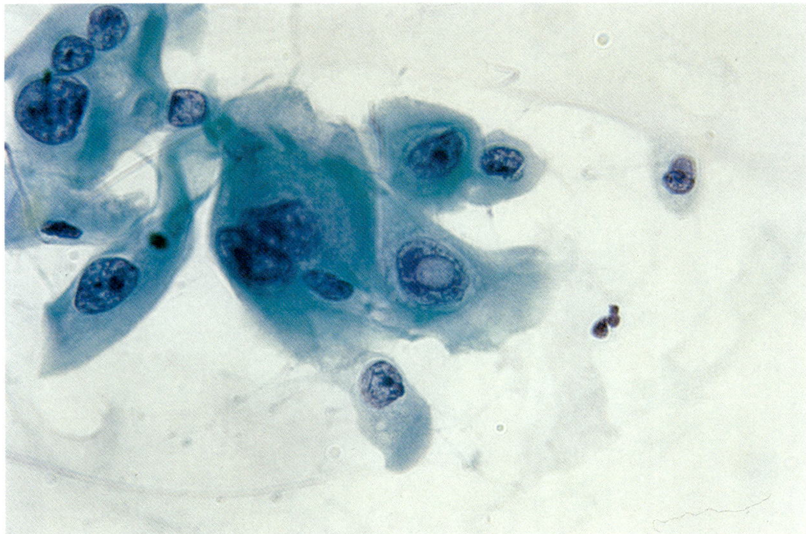

Fig. 67 Degenerated columnar epithelial cells following radiotherapy in a brushing cytology specimen. Enlargement of cytoplasms and nuclei and nuclear vacuolization are seen. Differentiation from malignant cells can be made on the basis of the terminal plates (arrows) and the resemblance to columnar cells. (X400, Pap.)

changes consist of vacuolation and abnormal enlargement of the nuclei and cytoplasm and the formation of prominent nucleoli. These changes are thought to be due to induction of cellular mutation and degeneration (Koss, 1979; Ono, 1981).

When injured bronchial epithelium is replaced by new epithelium after certain kinds of therapy, these cells show a pavement pattern of arrangement and possess an abundance of cytoplasm, round nuclei and prominent nucleoli. The chromatin

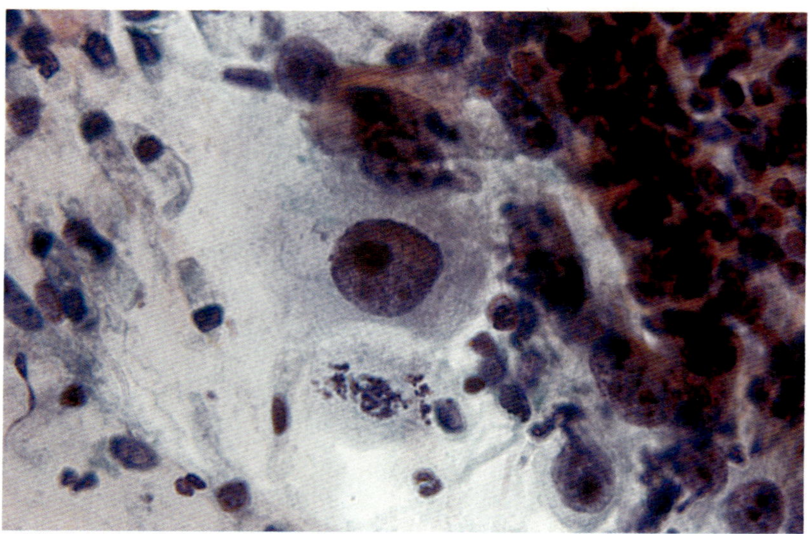

Fig. 68 Cells in a brushing specimen obtained following combined radio-and chemotherapy in a case of oat cell carcinoma show hyperchromasia and prominent nucleoli. Terminal plates (arrows) show distinction from malignant cells. (X400, Pap.)

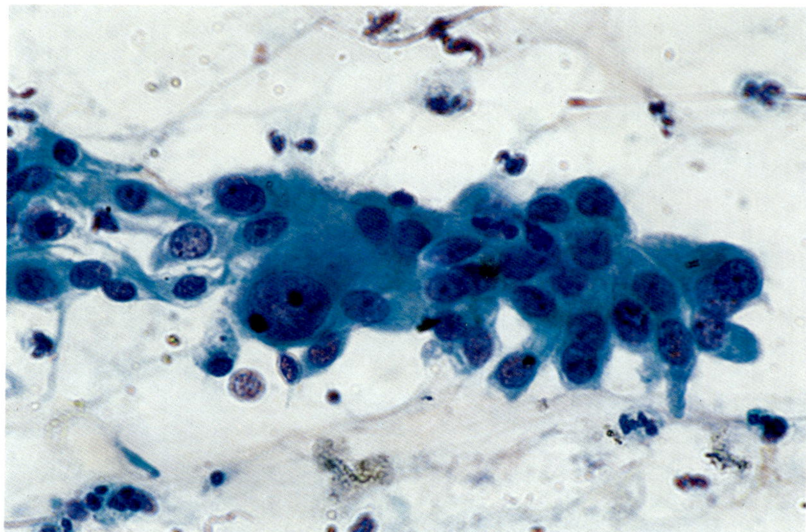

Fig. 69 Repair cells after hematoporphyrin derivative-laser photoradiation therapy. This brushing cytology specimen contains elongated cells with abundant cytoplasm. Nuclei show variation in size and the chromatin is finely granular. (X400, Pap.)

is finely granular (Fig. 69). These features resemble the characteristics of reserve cells in the female genital tract or metaplastic cells.

NONEPITHELIAL CELLS

Abnormal Histiocytes

Transformation of histiocytes, multinucleation and transfiguration are occasionally observed in pathologic conditions of the respiratory tract, such as inflammation and irritation due to the presence of foreign bodies.

Epithelioid cells are most frequently recognized in specimens, particularly those obtained by needle cytology, from patients with granulomatous lesions, such as tuberculosis and sarcoidosis. When epithelioid cells are recognized in sputum specimens, they are usually seen as isolated cells (Fig. 70). In specimens obtained by needle cytology, they often appear in clusters (Fig. 71). The cells have elongated cytoplasm, with bent, clear nuclei. In specimens obtained by either method, Langhans'-type giant cells (Fig. 72), which possess multiple nuclei located peripherally in a semicircular arrangement, are often found in the vicinity of the epithelioid cells (Nasiell et al., 1972).

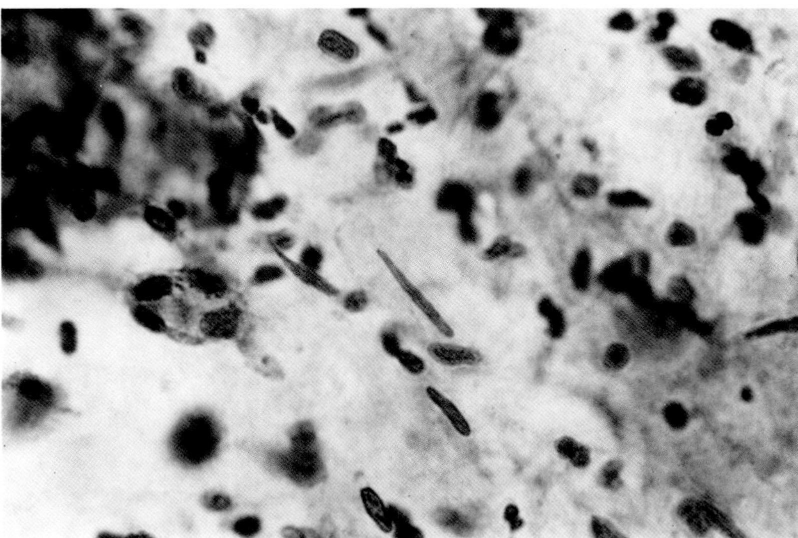

Fig. 70 Epitheloid cells in a sputum cytology preparation. Solitary epitheloid cells can be seen distributed throughout the specimen. These cells are characterized by spindle shaped cytoplasm with an elongated nucleus (from pulmonary tuberculosis). (X400, Pap.)

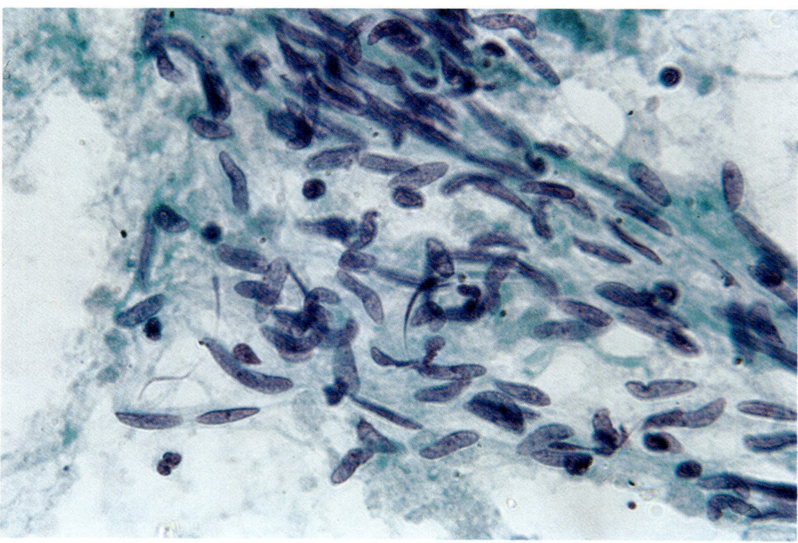

Fig. 71 Epitheloid cells in a needle aspiration cytology specimen in a case of tuberculosis. Numerous epitheloid cells with elongated or bent nuclei are seen in a case of tuberculosis. (X400, Pap.)

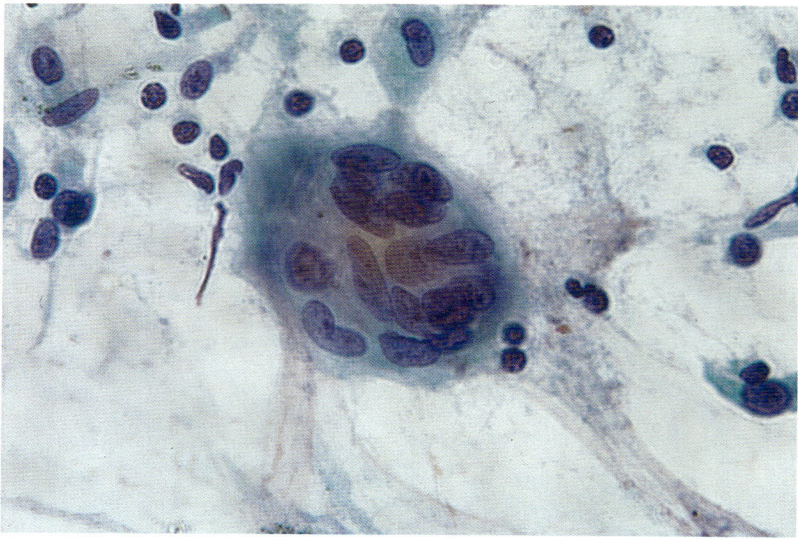

Fig. 72 Langhans' giant cells in a needle cytology specimen have finely granular chromatin. This cell was obtained from a case of tuberculosis. (X400, Pap.)

NONCELLULAR ELEMENTS

Charcot-Leyden Crystals

These crystals are most frequently seen in sputum specimens from patients with asthma and are believed to represent crystallized fragments of destroyed eosinophils. An increased number of eosinophils is often seen in the vicinity of these crystals (Fig. 73).

Curschmann's Spirals

These spirals are thought to be formed when mucin is excreted from the terminal bronchioles. Curschmann's spirals are frequently seen in obstructive lung diseases. Their central axes stain by hematoxylin and are surrounded by mucus sheath. They can appears as stringlike processes, spirals or coils (Fig. 74).

Asbestos Bodies

These bodies are frequently encountered in sputum specimens from asbestos workers. They resemble sticks of bamboo. Since a relationship between asbestos and lung cancer and malignant mesothelioma has been shown (W.H.O., 1973), the finding of asbestos bodies is extremely important (Fig. 75).

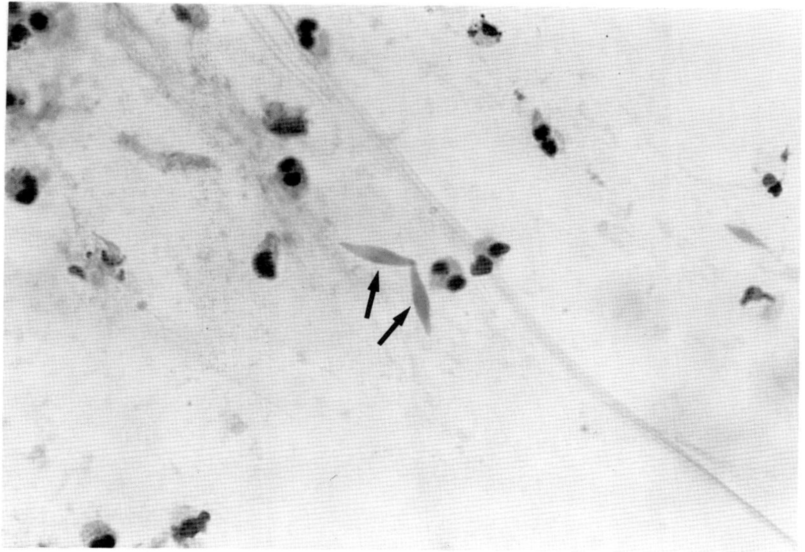

Fig. 73 Charcot-Leyden crystals (arrow) in a sputum cytology specimen. Octahedral crystals are characteristic. These crystals were observed in a case of asthma. (X400, Pap.)

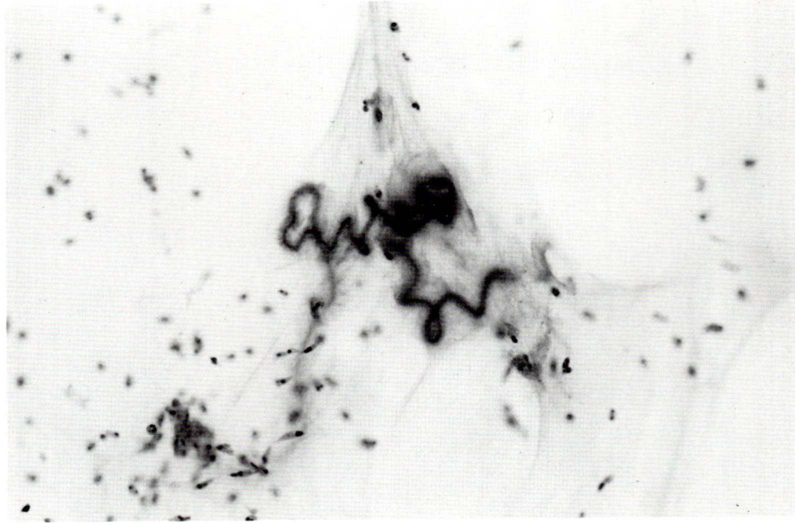

Fig. 74 Curschmann's spirals in a sputum cytology specimen. String-like processes, spirals or coils are characteristic (from chronic bronchitis). (X400, Pap.)

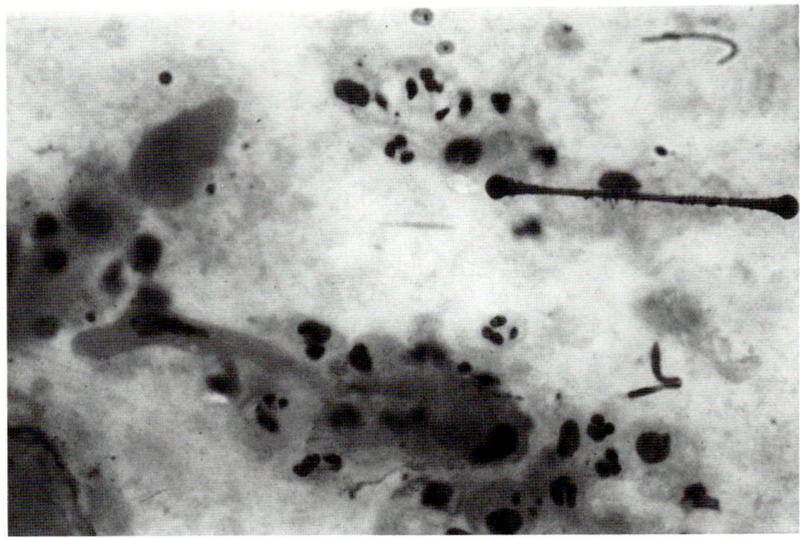

Fig. 75 Asbestos body in a sputum cytology specimen. The stick-like body suggests asbestosis. (X400, Pap.)

Candida Albicans

This fungus can be seen in sputum specimens from critically ill cases such as terminal cancer patients (Fig. 76). It resembles yeast and has long pseudohyphae. However, culture is necessary for a definitive diagnosis.

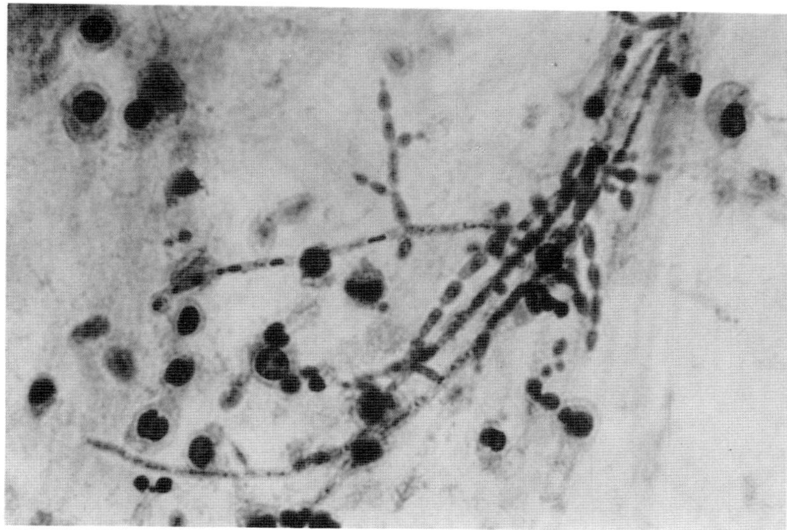

Fig. 76 Candida albicans in a sputum cytology specimen. The form of the Candida albicans in this sputum cytology specimen is described as yeast form or long pseudohyphae. (X400, Pap.)

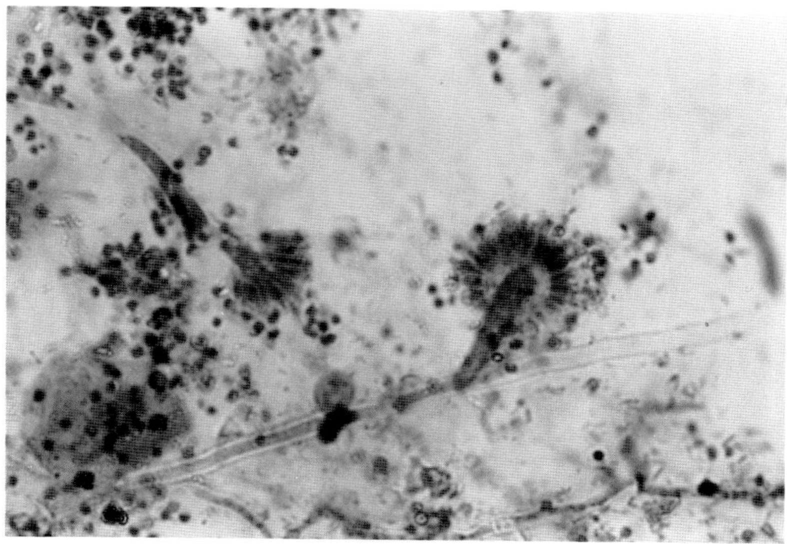

Fig. 77 Aspergillus in a needle aspiration cytology specimen from a case with pulmonary aspergillosis. (X400, Pap.)

Aspergillus

This fungus is often found in bronchial brushing materials and needle biopsy cytology specimens from patients with aspergilloma and in sputum specimens from patients with low immunocompetence (Fig. 77). Hyphae at an angle of 45 degrees and thick septa are characteristic features of this fungus.

Alternaria

This fungus can intrude during specimen preparation. It has no pathologic implications (Fig. 78).

Pneumocystis Carinii

P. carinii is a parasite that is most often seen in cases of renal transplantation or in newborn infants. Current thinking is that patients with reduced immunocompetence are susceptible to infections caused by this parasite. Specimens are stained with methenamine silver or by the Gram-Weigert method (Fig. 79) (Oiwa et al., 1980).

Vegetable Cells

Many food cells are recognized in sputum specimens. They occasionally resemble cancer cells. Figure 80 shows a vegetable cell observed in a sputum specimen from a patient who had eaten pimentos. The findings resemble those of squamous cell carcinoma. In another patient who had consumed fermented soybeans, the vegetable cell that was recognized in the sputum specimen showed a strong resemblance to adenocarcinoma cells (Fig. 81). Cells of a kind of seaweed (laver) occasionally resemble those of small cell carcinoma (Fig. 82). Food cells encountered naturally depend on the dietary habits of each patient.

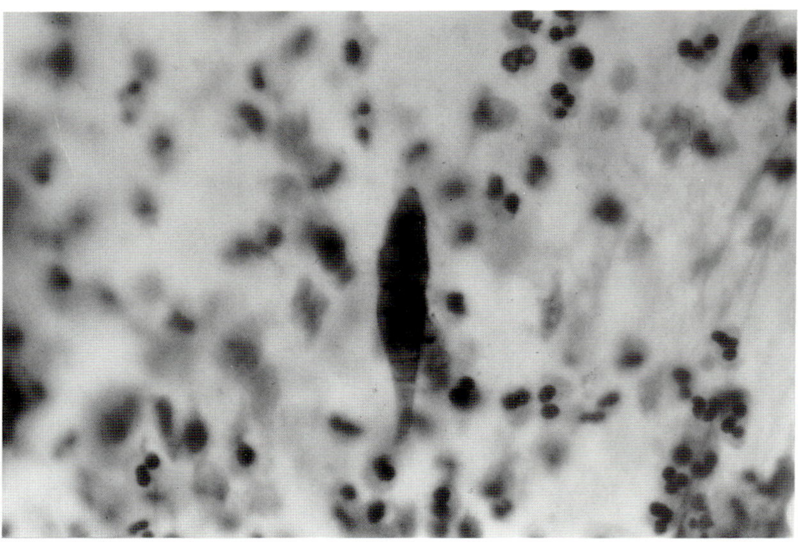

Fig. 78 Alternaria in a sputum cytology specimen. It is spindle shaped and the bands are characteristic. (X400, Pap.)

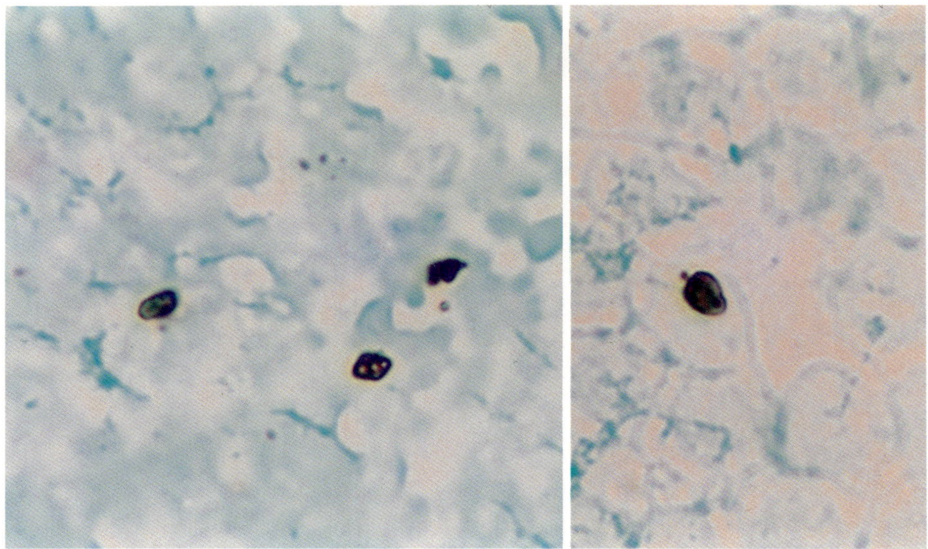

Fig. 79 Pneumocystis carinii in a needle biopsy cytology specimen. The tiny round organisms are 4—5 μ in size. (X400, Pap.)

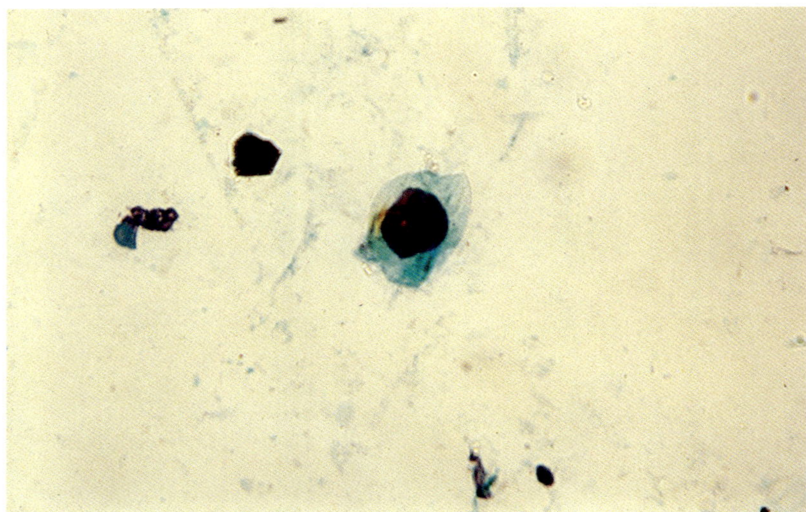

Fig. 80 Vegetable cell (pimento) in a sputum cytology specimen. These cells can be misdiagnosed as squamous cell carcinoma cells. (X400, Pap.)

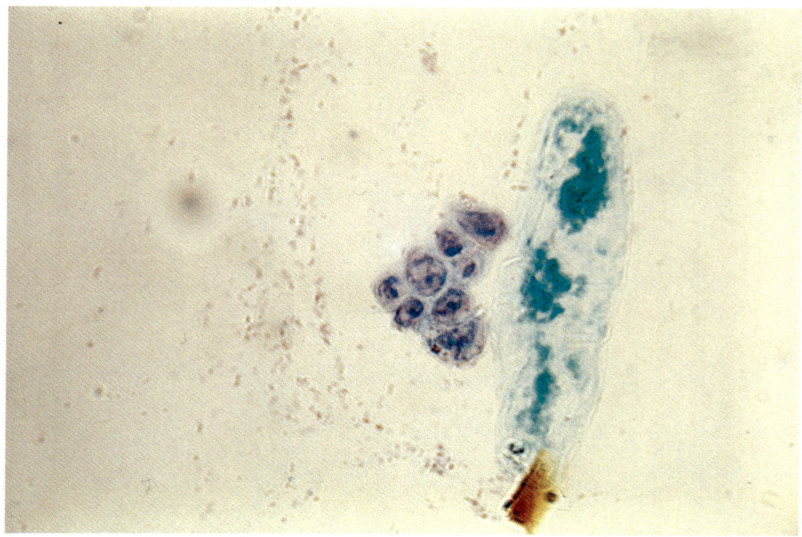

Fig. 81 Vegetable cells (soybean) in a sputum cytology specimen. These cells show resemblance to adenocarcinoma. (X400, Pap.)

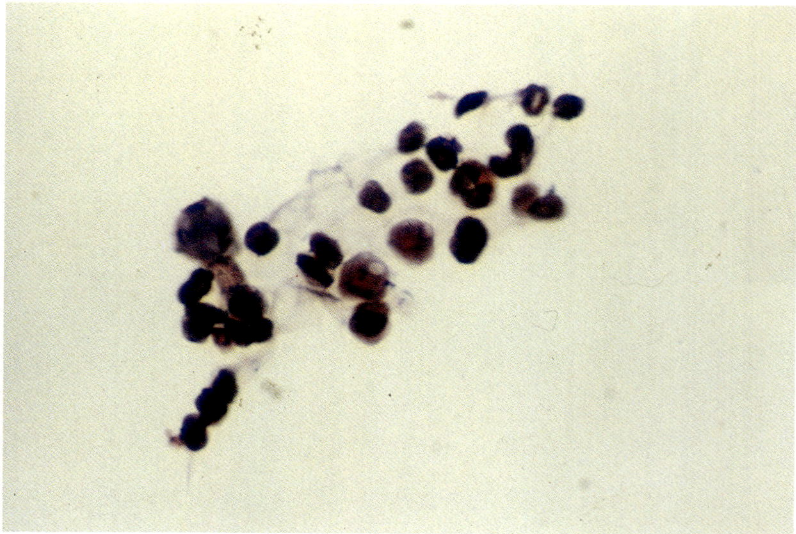

Fig. 82 Vegetable cells (kelp) in a sputum cytology specimen. Cells of some kinds of seaweed resemble small cell carcinoma. (X400, Pap.)

BENIGN TUMORS

Benign tumors of the bronchus or lung are rare in comparison to lung cancer. Oldham (1980) recently published a classification of benign tumors (Table 10), and of these hamartoma is the most common.

These tumors do not exfoliate in sputum but transthoracic needle and TBAC techniques are effective methods to obtain materials. Apart from neurogenic tumors the cells show little atypia. The cellular appearance is close to that of the tissue from which they derive. Some show calcification. Hamartoma and neurilemmoma are presented here as representative cases.

Table 10 Benign Tumors of the Lung and Bronchus
(from Oldham, Jr., H.N.: Surg. Clin. North Amer., 60: 825—834, 1980)

Epithelial Tumors	d. granular cell myoblastoma
1. Papilloma	e. leiomyoma
2. Polyp	f. neurogenic tumors
Mesodermal Tumors	Developmental Tumors
1. Vascular	1. Hamartoma
a. hemangioma	a. chondromatous hamartoma
b. lymphangioma	b. blastoma
c. hemangiopericytoma	2. Teratoma
2. Bronchial	3. Clear cell ("sugar") tumor
a. fibroma	Inflammatory Pseudotumors
b. chondroma	1. Plasma cell tumor
c. lipoma	2. Xanthoma

Hamartoma

The most common type is hamartochondroma. Generally hamartoma tissue can be seen to contain cartilage, connective tissue, fatty tissue and columnar epithelium, but occasionally cartilage is not recognized.

This tumor usually arises in the periphery of the lungs and is hard. It is difficult to obtain hamartoma cells by bronchial brushing or expectoration of sputum. It is possible to diagnose this tumor on the basis of cell features, such as their fibrous nature, the presence of clusters of spindle cells without nuclear atypia and the occasional appearance of cartilaginous cells. Hamartoma cells can be obtained by percutaneous needle cytology (TMC needle) or by transbronchial aspiration cytology techniques (Fig. 83) (Bateson and Abott, 1960; Dahlgren, 1966; Ramzy, 1976).

Neurilemmoma (Schwannoma)

This tumor develops generally in the chest wall and the mediastinum, but is extremely rare in the lung. Neurilemmoma cells show marked atypia, namely variation in size and shape of their nuclei (Fig. 84).

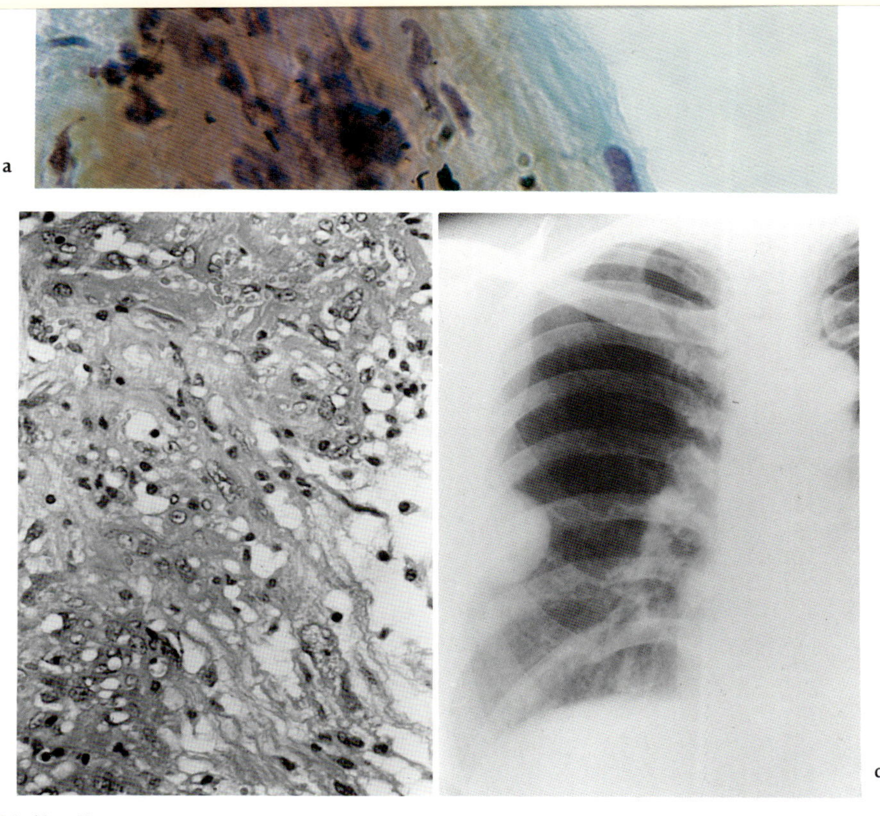

Fig. 84 Neurilemmoma
(a)   Needle cytology specimen. These cells reveal a bizarre shape with strong atypia. Chromatin is finely granular and proliferative. (X400, Pap.)
(b)   Histologic findings. The cells with abundant cytoplasm and bizarre nuclei show solid proliferation. (X200, H.E.)
(c)   Chest X-ray findings showing a round tumor shadow in the chest wall.

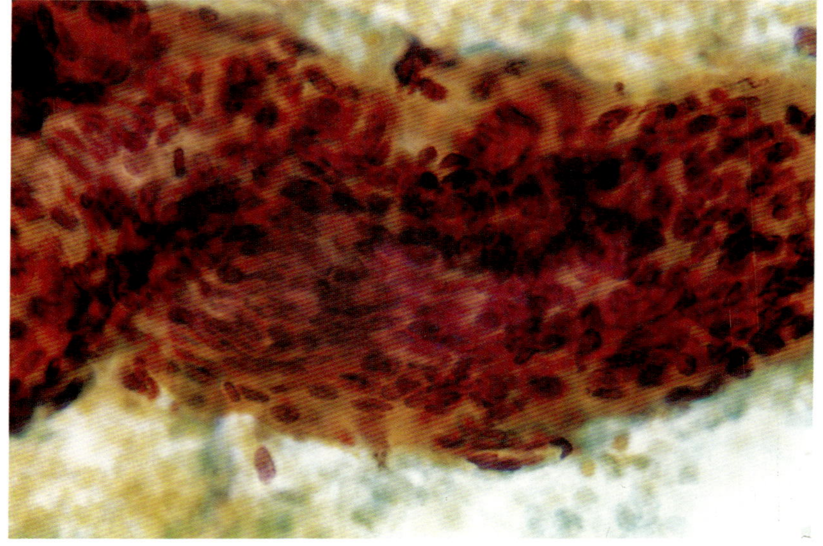

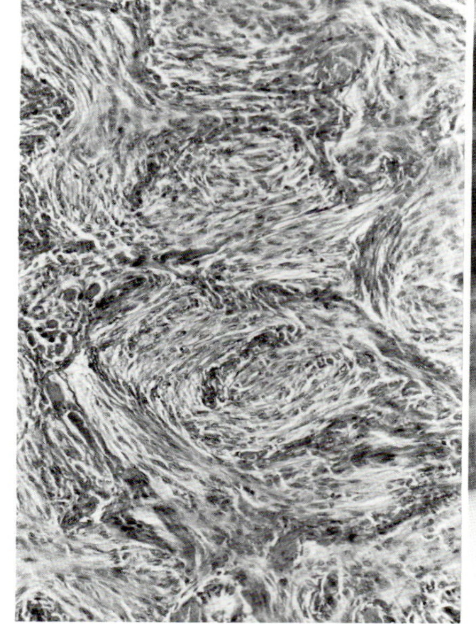

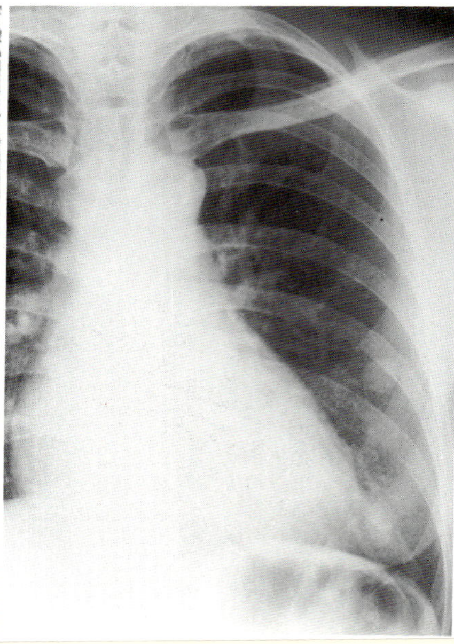

V

Squamous Metaplasia

There are two theories concerning the origin of squamous metaplasia, direct and indirect development. The theory of the direct origin of squamous metaplasia is that transfiguration occurs directly from mature epithelium, such as ciliated columnar cells, whereas the theory of indirect origin suggests that cellular transformation occurs from immature cells, such as basal cells or reserve cells (Nasiell, 1963). The latter is most probable in the respiratory tract. Squamous metaplasia can occur easily when the epithelium is injured by various conditions or agents, such as inflammation, exposure to carcinogens and metabolic disturbance. Squamous metaplasia arises after several cellular changes, such as exfoliation of columnar cells, goblet cell hyperplasia, slit formation and basal cell hyperplasia (Nasiell, 1968). It appears that squamous metaplasia is an initial manifestation of the body's defense mechanism against noxious stimuli (Kato et al., 1977, 1982c; Konaka et al., 1982b. Ono et al., 1982). Squamous metaplasia can show varying degrees of atypia, which have been divided into four categories according to the degree of nuclear atypia (Saccomanno et al., 1974; Kato et al., 1977, 1982c; Nasiell, 1966; Konaka et al., 1982a). The categories are nonatypical, mildly atypical, moderately atypical and severely atypical. Squamous metaplasia shows a pavement pattern of cellular arrangement. The nucleus-to-cytoplasm ratio is relatively high. Individual cells show nuclei a little larger than those of basal cells. The cytoplasm stains strongly, occasionally with an orange-ophilic staining pattern. Variation in the size of nuclei, distribution of chromatin, aggregation of chromatin, amount of cytoplasm and degree of cellular adherence depend on the degree of atypia.

DEGREE OF ATYPIA

The categorization of the degree of atypia of squamous metaplasia is based on the work of Nasiell and coworkers (1978) (Table 11) and Saccomanno (1974, 1978) (Table 12) on sputum cytology specimens. However, the appearance of fresh cells obtained by brushing technique via the fiberoptic bronchoscope is slightly different from the appearance of cells in sputum specimens. Table 13 shows the classification of the degree of atypia of fresh cells as made by the authors (Kato et al., 1978b). The reason for the difference is that cells in sputum that have been exfoliated show a relatively high degree of degeneration. Cells in sputum specimens are smaller than those in brushing specimens. In sputum specimens, the greater the degree of atypia, the greater the tendency for cells to appear singly. Conversely, in brushing specimens, the cells usually appear in clusters due to the

Table 11 Criteria of the grade of atypia in squamous metaplasia.

(summarized from Nasiell, M., Kato, H., Auer, G., et al.: Cancer, 1511–1521, 1978)

Squamous metaplasia without atypia
1. Nuclei are round or slightly oval.
2. The chromatin is finely granular.
3. The nuclear size is similar to that of the oral squamous cells or somewhat larger.
4. Single cells are rare.

Squamous metaplasia with mild atypia
1. The nuclear size is slightly variable.
2. There is usually a slight hyperchromasia in a few cells in these cell clusters which otherwise exhibit the same general character as non-atypical metaplastic cells.
3. Single metaplastic cells are rare.

Squamous metaplasia with moderate atypia
1. Several nuclei in the cell clusters show variation in size and chromatin staining intensity.
2. Some nuclei show distinct hyperchromasia, though the chromatin is usually finely granular.
3. Single atypical metaplastic cells may occur.

Squamous metaplasia with severe atypia
1. There is a distinct variation in nuclear shape.
2. Nuclear hyperchromasia is a striking feature.
3. The nuclear membrane may be irregular and the chromatin may be coarse.
4. There are usually a few single metaplastic cells with severely nuclear atypia.
5. The metaplastic character is, however, retained, i.e. the abnormality of the single metaplastic cells is not as pronounced as in carcinoma.

Table 12 Cytological criteria for squamous cell metaplasia.

(from Saccomanno, G.: Diagnostic Pulmonary Cytology, American Society of Clinical Pathologists, Chicago, 1978)

Regular Metaplasia

1. Cells all of about same size.
2. Nuclei of same size with regular nuclear/cytoplasmic ratio.
3. Nuclear material fine and powdery with rare chromocenter.
4. Cytoplasm usually basophilic.
5. Cells usually occur in sheets, but may be single.

Metaplasia, Mild Atypia

1. Cells vary slightly in size.
2. Nuclei vary slightly in size, and nuclear/cytoplasmic ratio may vary slightly.
3. Nuclear material still fine and powdery with rare clusters of nuclear material near the nuclear membrane.
4. Cytoplasm may be acidophilic.
5. Cells usually occur in sheets, but may be found singly.

Metaplasia, Moderate Atypia

1. Cells vary moderately in size; some are smaller but most are larger than in mild metaplasia.
2. Nuclei vary significantly in size with moderate variation in nuclear/cytoplasmic ratio.
3. Nuclear material is still fine and powdery in most areas, but nuclear masses are abundant, particularly along the membrane.
4. Nuclear lobulations, crevices, and nodules are present.
5. Cytoplasm may be basophilic, but acidophilia predominates.
6. Cells usually occur in sheets, but an increase in single cells is found.

Metaplasia, Marked Atypia

1. Cells vary markedly in size, but are generally larger than the moderate atypias.
2. Nuclear pleomorphism is marked, and nuclear material is coarse and sometimes clustered about the nuclear membrane. Nuclear/cytoplasmic ratio varies, with extremes.
3. Nucleoli are present but are small and may be acidophilic.
4. Acidophilic cytoplasm predominates.
5. Single cells predominate.

Table 13 Cytomorphology of squamous metaplasia in brushing specimens

---

Regular squamous metaplasia
1. Cells occur mainly in clusters with good cellular adherence. Single cells are rare. Cellular arrangement is flat, pavement-like and overlapping is rare.
2. Cellular shape is polygonal, cuboidal or occasionally round and the size is uniform.
3. Cytoplasm stains light green (cyanophilic, basophilic).
4. Nuclear shape is round or oval and the size is almost the same as or a little larger in columnar cells and there are no variations.
5. The nuclear membrane is regular and thin.
6. Chromatin is finely granular.
7. Nucleoli, when present, are very small and round but usually are absent.
8. The N/C ratio is small and constant.

Mildly atypical squamous metaplasia
1. Cells occur mainly in clusters with good cellular adherence. Single cells are rare. Cellular arrangement is pavement-like and cells overlap slightly on occasion.
2. The cellular shape is polygonal, cuboidal or occasionally round and the size is slightly variable.
3. Cytoplasm stains green.
4. The nuclear shape is round or oval, and size varies slightly.
5. The nuclear membrane is regular and thin.
6. Chromatin is finely granular and some nuclei show hyperchromasia.
7. Nucleoli are small, round and generally present.
8. The N/C ratio varies slightly.

Moderately atypical squamous metaplasia
1. Cells occur in clusters. Cellular arrangment is pavement-like and cellular overlapping occurs. Single cells may occur.
2. The cellular shape is polygonal and the size varies.
3. The cytopalsm stains light green distrinctly and is occasionally eosinophilic.
4. The nuclear shape is round or oval and size varies.
5. The nuclear membrane is generally regular and thin but is occasionally irregular.
6. The chromatin is granular and hyperchromatic.
7. There is generally a single nucleolus which is comparatively large and irregular.
8. The N/C ratio is variable.

Severely atypical squamous metaplasia
1. Cells still occur in clusters and show pavement-like arrangement. Cellular overlapping is distinct. Single cells occur frequently.
2. The cellular shape is polygonal and distinct variation in size can be seen.
3. The cytoplasm distinctly stains light green with a dark eosinophilic stain on occasion.
4. Nuclear shape vary distinctly and are irregular. A striking variation in nuclear size can be seen.
5. The nuclear membrane is thin but may be irregular and thickened.
6. Chromatin is granular, and on occasion coarse. Striking hyperplasia is recognized.
7. Nucleoli are large and irregular but are unclear in hyperchromatic nuclei.
8. The N/C ratio is generally large.
9. Most cells in clusters satisfy only some of these criteria.

---

nature of the harvesting method. However, in brushing specimens, the amount of cellular overlapping increases in accordance with the increased degree of atypia. The cytoplasm of cells observed in sputum specimens is frequently orangeophilic, whereas the cytoplasm usually stains light green in brushings specimens. The chromatin in sputum specimens shows great variability in appearance, from finely granular to coarsely granular or homogeneous, whereas brushing specimens show either finely or coarsely granular chromatin. Nucleoli are rarely observed in sputum cytology specimens, whereas they are frequently seen in brushing cytology specimens. In the latter, the nucleoli are extremely small in cases with a low degree of atypia, but as the degree of atypia increases, the nucleoli show a tendency to increase in size (Figs. 85—89).

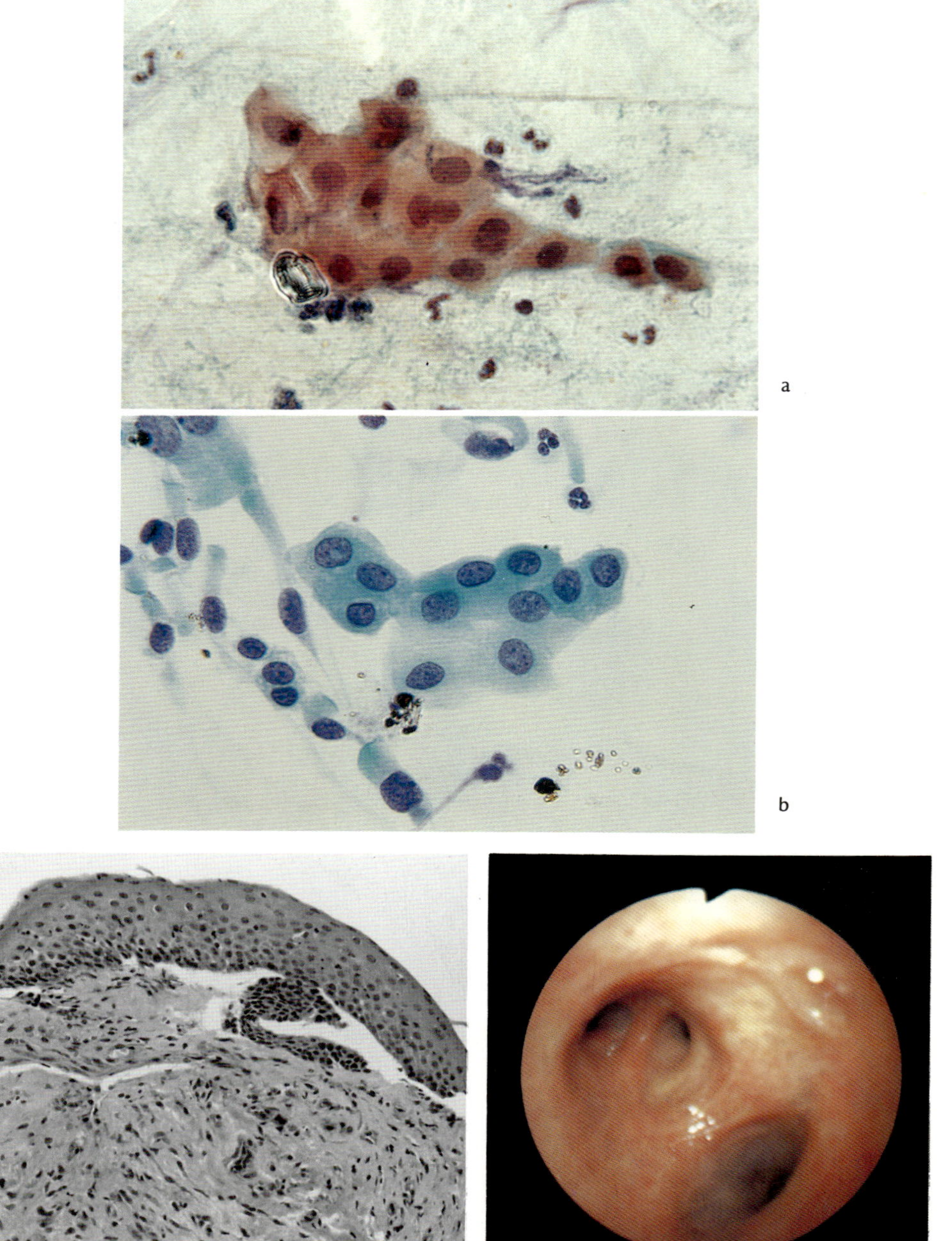

Fig. 85 Squamous metaplasia without nuclear atypia. These specimens were obtained from a patient
with chronic bronchitis.
(a)   Sputum cytology specimen. Nuclei are round or oval, and chromatin is finely granular. (X400,
       Pap.)
(b)   Brushing cytology specimen. Cells appear in a cluster. Chromatin is finely granular. Nuclei are a
       little larger than those of ciliated columnar cells. (X400, Pap.)
(c)   Bronchoscopic biopsy specimen. Non-atypical cells are arranged regularly. (X100, H.E.)
(d)   Bronchoscopic findings. Bronchial mucosa shows slight redness at the bifurcation of the left
       upper lobe and lower lobe bronchi. The endoscopic findings of non-atypical squamous metaplasia
       sometimes show no abnormalities.

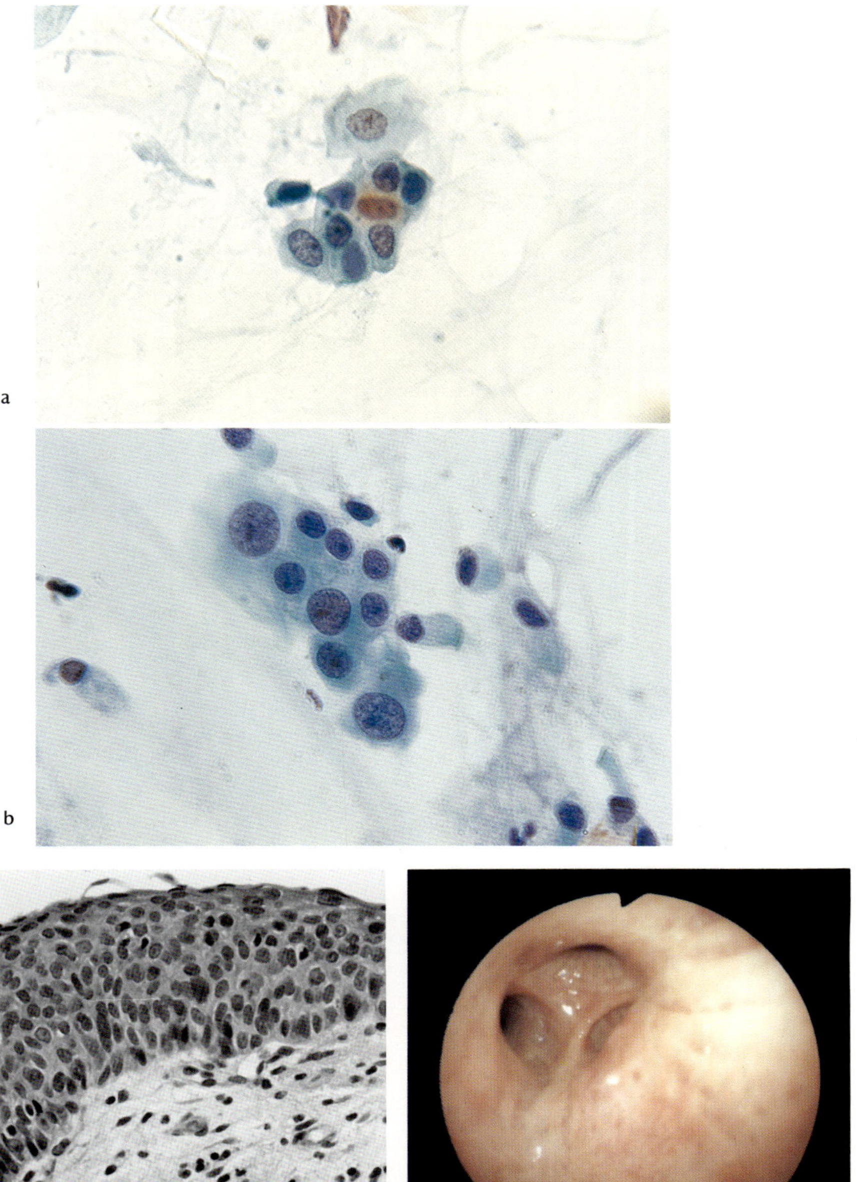

Fig. 86 Squamous metaplasia with mild nuclear atypia. These specimens were obtained from a smoker.
(a) Sputum cytology specimen. The nuclear size is slightly variable and chromatin is finely granular. (X400, Pap.)
(b) Brushing cytology specimen. The cytoplasm stains light blue green and the nuclear size is variable. Chromatin is fine and nucleoli are recognizable. (X400, Pap.)
(c) Bronchoscopic biopsy specimen. The thickened mucosa consists of the cells with slight variation in size. (X200, H.E.)
(d) Bronchoscopic findings showing slight thickness and redness of the mucosa of the bifurcation between the right upper lobe bronchus and the truncus intermedius.

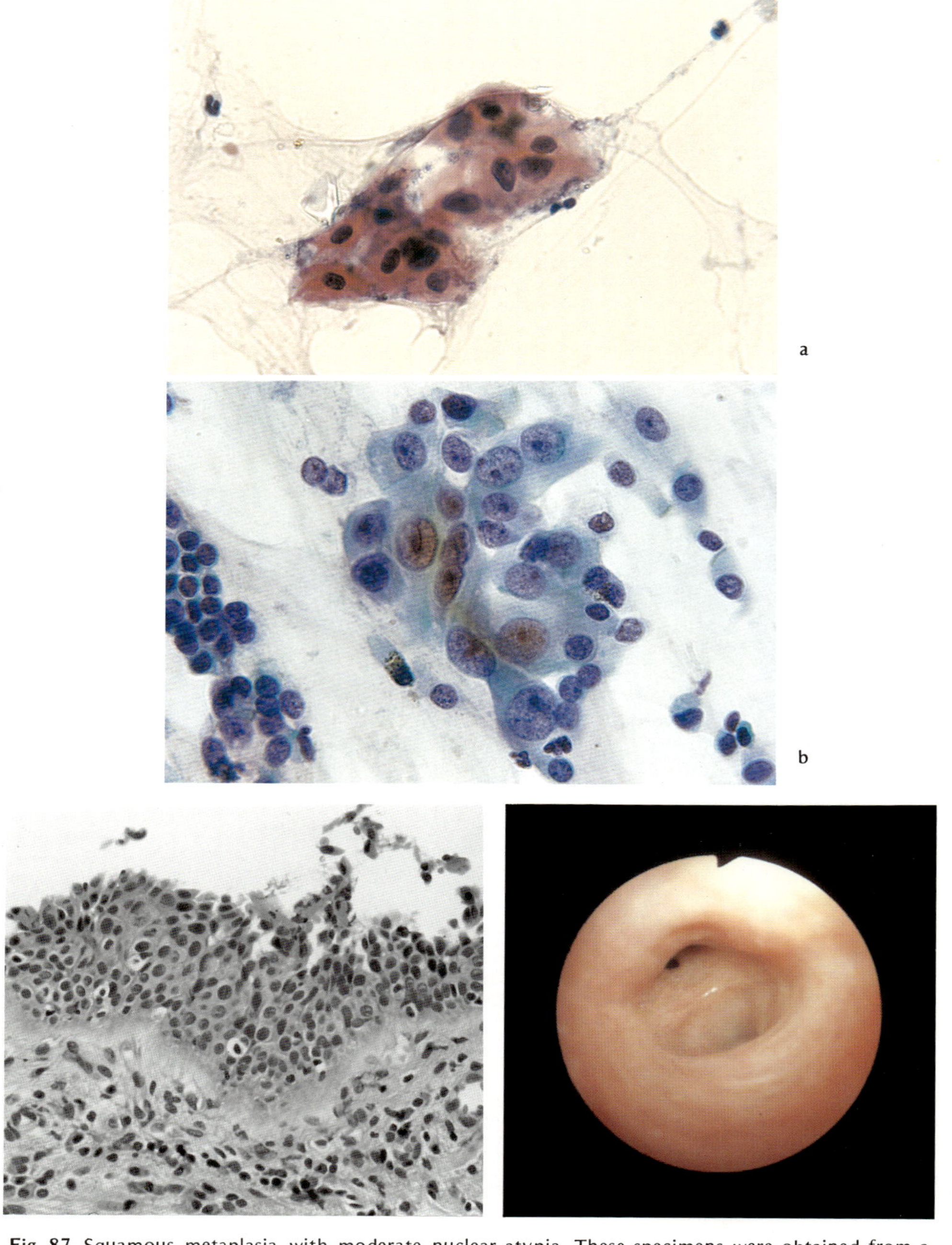

Fig. 87 Squamous metaplasia with moderate nuclear atypia. These specimens were obtained from a patient with pulmonary tuberculosis.
(a)   Sputum cytology specimen. Nuclei show variations in size. Some nuclei show hyperchromasia and the cytoplasm is eosinophilic. (X400, Pap.)
(b)   Bronchoscopic brushing specimen. Cytoplasm is basophilic. The nuclear size is large in comparison to adjacent columnar cells. Hyperchromasia is not striking. Nucleoli are prominent. (X400, Pap.)
(c)   Bronchoscopic biopsy specimen. Cells with prominent nucleoli are arranged irregularly. (X200, H.E.)
(d)   Bronchoscopic findings show thickening of the mucosa of the left upper lobe bronchus.

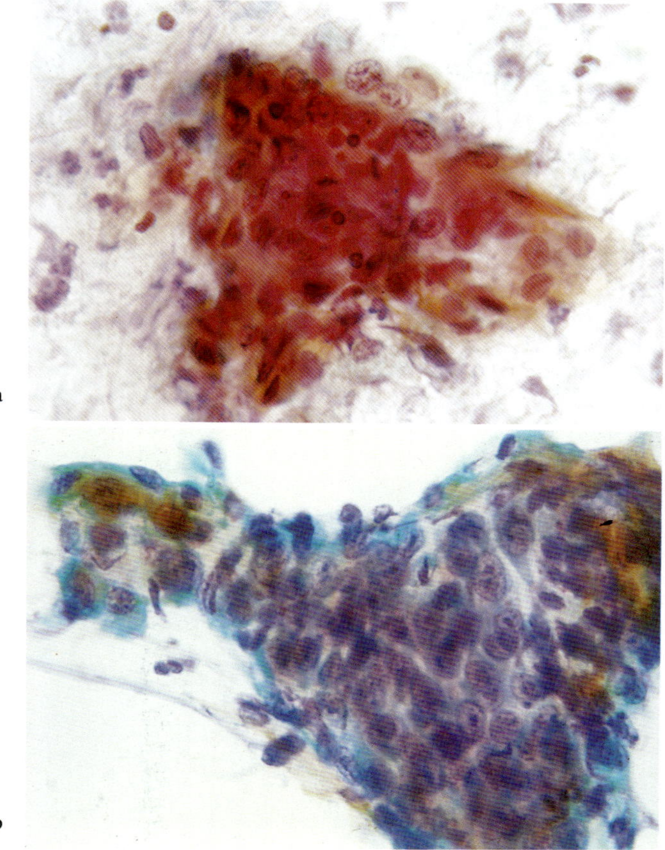

Fig. 88 Squamous metaplasia with severely nuclear atypia. These specimens were obtained from a heavy smoker.
(a) Sputum cytology specimen. The nuclear shape varies distinctly. Some nuclei show hyperchromasia. The nuclear membrane is irregular and nucleoli are seen. (X400, Pap.)
(b) Brushing cytology specimen. A large cluster is seen. Some cells with prominent nucleoli overlap each other. Cytoplasms stain basophilic. (X400, Pap.)

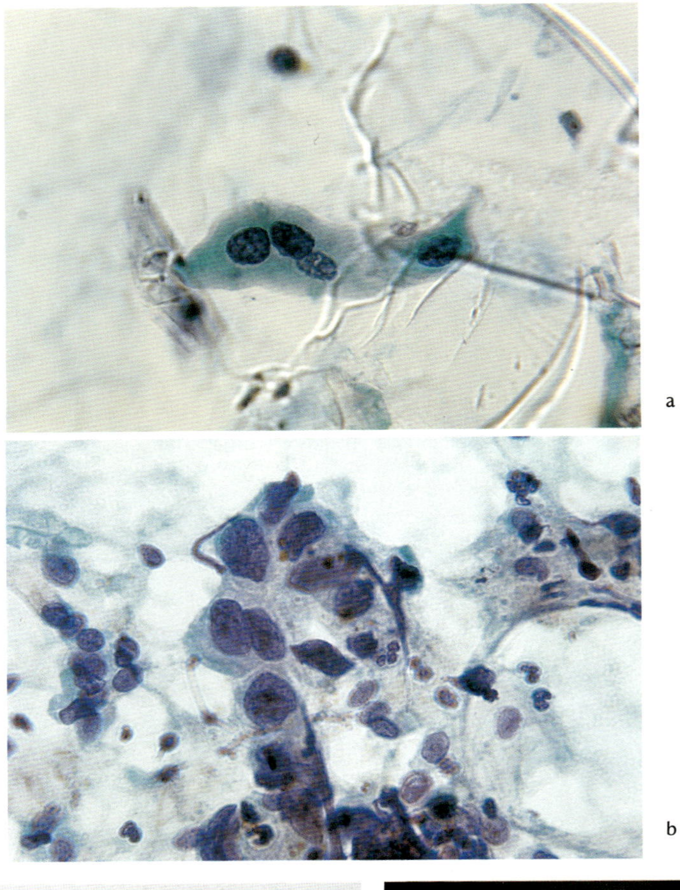

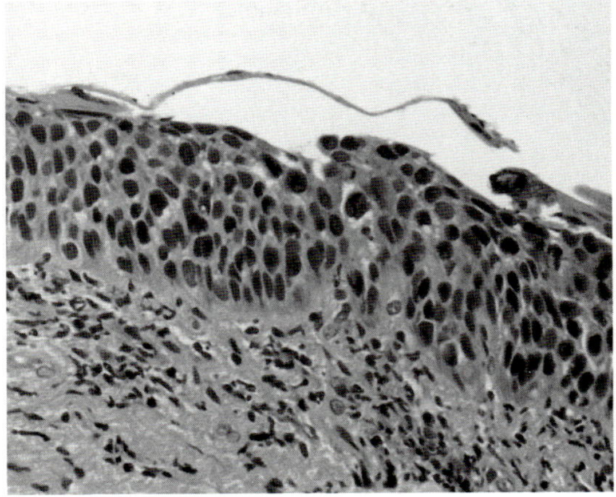

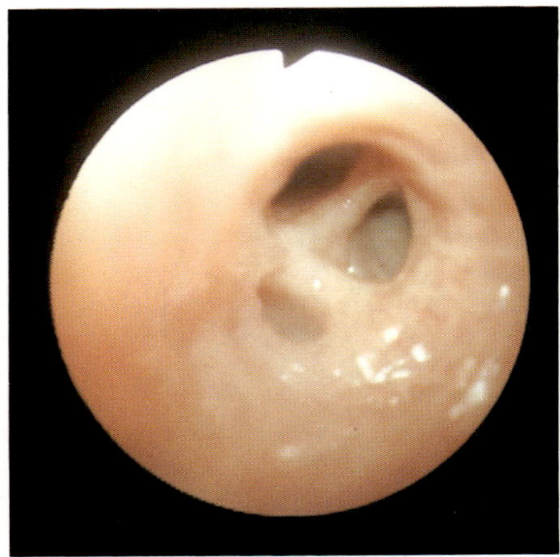

Fig. 89 Squamous metaplasia with severely nuclear atypia. These specimens were obtained from a heavy smoker.

(a) Sputum cytology specimen. Striking hyperchromasia, coarse chromatin and irregular nuclear membrane are seen. (X400, Pap.)

(b) Brushing cytology specimen. Enlargement of nuclear size, hyperchromasia, prominent nucleoli are seen. Cytoplasms stain basophilic. (X400, Pap.)

(c) Bronchial biopsy specimen. Irregularly shaped nuclei with coarse chromatin are arranged irregularly. (X200, H.E.)

(d) Bronchoscopic findings. Bronchial mucosa show irregularity at the bifurcation of the left upper division bronchi.

IN COMBINATION WITH SQUAMOUS CELL CARCINOMA

As has been stated earlier, the pathologic development of squamous cell carcinoma of the lung in human beings is poorly understood. The report by Saccomanno and coworkers in 1974 is representative of several claims that squamous cell carcinoma develops from squamous metaplasia. However, other authors (Oota, 1955; Melamed et al., 1977) have postulated that squamous cell carcinoma develops from normal bronchial epithelium on the basis of the finding that intraepithelial squamous cell carcinoma, including cases of microscopic invasion, can be observed in the absence of squamous metaplasia in surrounding areas in some cases. But these pathologic findings on which these contentions were based derived in many cases only from surgical or autopsy specimens. It is probable that the absence of squamous metaplasia beside squamous cell carcinoma is the result of replacement growth of intraepithelial carcinoma (Takahashi, 1981). Until the study by the authors and their colleagues, there was no well-documented report of a large animal experimental series elucidating the pathogenic process of bronchogenic carcinoma. In practice, it is extremely difficult to distinguish cellular development during the clinical course.

Therefore, to elucidate the pathogenetic process in specific local sites, the authors established an experimental carcinogenesis model in large animals that could be followed endoscopically (Hayata et al., 1977; Kato et al., 1977, 1980b; Konaka et al., 1982). The carcinogen, 20-methylcholanthrene (20-MC), was selected on the basis of a review of the literature, and mongrel dogs and beagles were used as laboratory animals. Preliminary work showed that 20-MC instilled into bronchi could cause peripheral lung cancer lesions in dogs, but these could not be followed endoscopically (Nakajima et al., 1975). The 20-MC was therefore administered via a catheter with a retractable needle developed by the authors at Tokyo Medical College Hospital for injection through fiberoptic endoscopes. The site of the injection was the bifurcation of the right apical and cardiac lode bronchi.

A variety of changes were observed to precede the development of squamous cell carcinoma, and the general process is summarized in Figures 90 and 91. Most of the squamous metaplasia that was observed during the carcinogenetic process in dogs was immature squamous metaplasia (transitional epithelioid metaplasia).

On the other hand, some investigators (Tipton, 1964; Saffiotti, 1967, 1969; Stenbäck, 1973; Schreiber, 1974; Marchok, 1975) believe that squamous metaplasia is a widespread phenomenon that can occur as a result of a variety of conditions and that it is not specifically related to squamous cell carcinoma (Niskanen, 1949). However, a study of lesions and their localization (Table 14) has revealed that the frequency of the occurrence of squamous metaplasia is significantly higher in the vicinity of squamous cell carcinoma lesions than in the vicinity of any other type of carcinoma (Kato et al., 1980c). Therefore, the authors believe that a relationship between squamous metaplasia and squamous cell carcinoma is possible.

Examination of the DNA content in specimens from cases of the various types of atypical squamous metaplasia, intraepithelial carcinoma and squamous cell

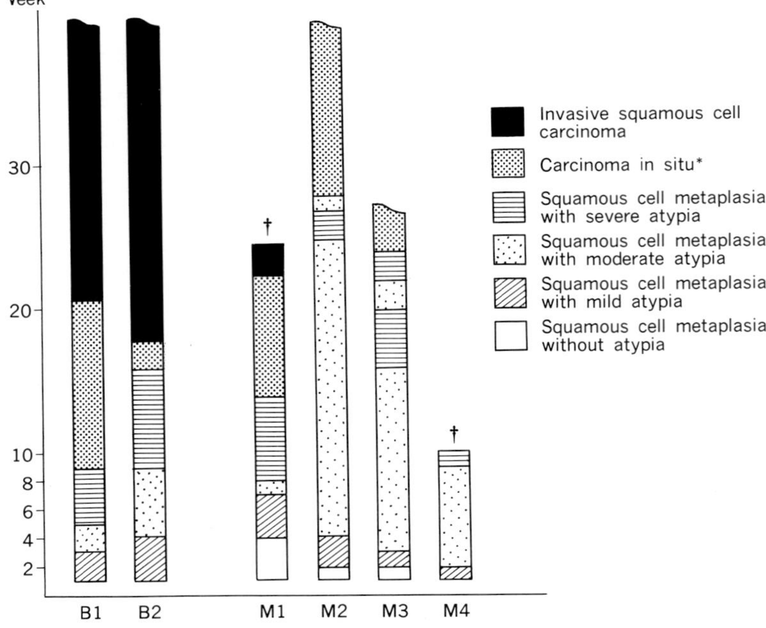

Fig. 90 Development of experimental lung cancer in dogs. Previously published in Kato, H. et al., 1980c.

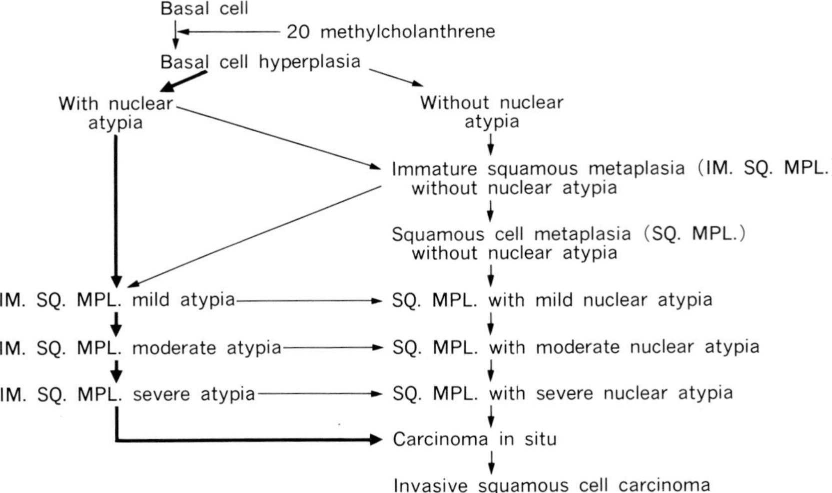

Fig. 91 Carcinogenetic process of experimental pulmonary squamous cell carcinoma in dogs.

Table 14 Frequency of Accompanying Squamous Metaplasia in the Vicinity of the Lesion According to Histologic Type

1) **Brushing Cytology Specimen:**

Histologic type	Cases	Squamous metaplasia	Atypical squamous metaplasia
Squamous cell carcinoma	31	24 (77.4%)	14 (45.2%)
Adenocarcinoma	25	12 (48.0%)	4 (16.0%)
Small cell carcinoma	11	4 (36.4%)	1 (9.0%)
Heavy smoker (>20/day)	100	29 (29.0%)	—

2) **Histologic Specimen:**

Histologic type	Cases	Squamous metaplasia	Atypical squamous metaplasia
Squamous cell carcinoma	23	15 (65.2%)	10 (43.5%)
Adenocarcinoma	27	9 (33.3%)	4 (14.8%)
Small cell carcinoma	4	1 (25.0%)	—

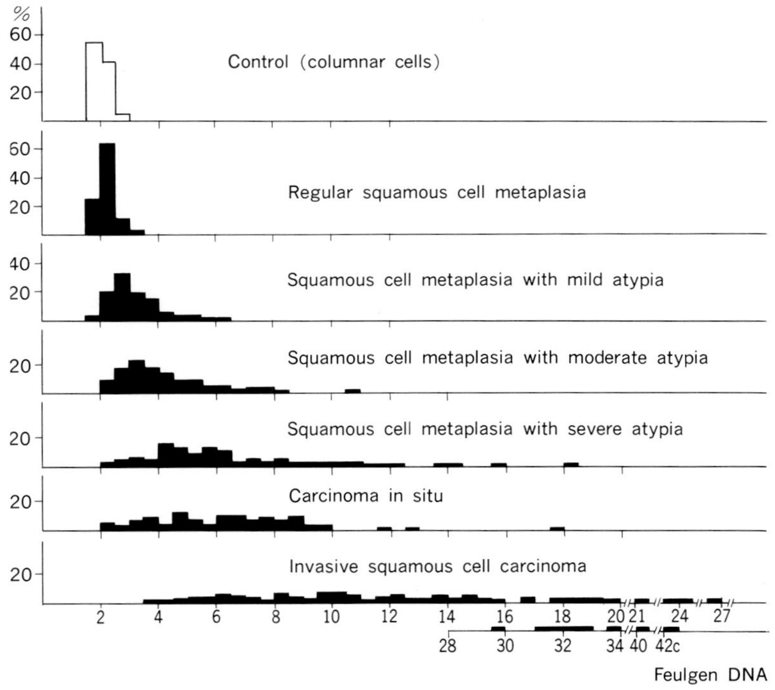

Fig. 92 Nuclear DNA histograms during the process from normal mucosa to invasive squamous carcinoma in dogs.

carcinoma revealed that as the degree of atypia increases, the amount of DNA increases and that this phenomenon is accompanied by changes in the histogram to a wide heteroploid distribution pattern (Fig. 92) (Kato et al., 1977; Nasiell et al., 1978). These findings indicate that a morphologic progression toward a malignant appearance is reflected by a cytochemical progression in that direction.

Although it has been suggested that there are two types of squamous metaplasia, namely, squamous metaplasia possessing a carcinogenetic potential, and that resulting from a toxic reaction (Kobayashi et al., 1978), we have been unable to discern any morphologic or cytochemical feature that would serve as a reliable basis for such a differentiation, and it is our impression that squamous metaplasia represents a single entity regardless of its origin or ultimate progression. Therefore, whether or not squamous metaplasia progresses to carcinoma appears to be the result of a variety of considerations, such as chronic exposure to a carcinogen and conditions affecting the host (nucleic acid abnormalities, histochemical abnormalities, disturbance of immunocompetence and metabolic or hormonal disorders).

On the basis of various lines of evidence, atypical squamous metaplasia can thus be considered to be possibly related to the carcinogenetic process in lung cancer. However, it should be remembered that not all squamous metaplasia should necessarily be considered as requiring close follow-up but, rather, that special attention should be given primarily to severely atypical squamous metaplasia.

We follow up squamous metaplasia as shown in Table 15.

Table 15 Following up of squamous metaplasia.

Squamous metaplastic atypia	Follow up
Regular squamous metaplasia Mildly atypical squamous metaplasia	Annual sputum cytologic examination
Moderately atypical squamous metaplasia	Semiannual sputum cytologic examination
Severely atypical squamous metaplasia	Sputum cytology + bronchoscopy every three months

VI

Malignant Tumor Cells

As a result of developments in lung cancer diagnostic methods, the cytologist encounters increasing numbers of fresh cytology specimens that are obtained by the fiberoptic bronchoscopic brushing technique or the percutaneous needle cytology technique. Before the development of the fiberoptic bronchoscope, almost all cytology specimens were sputum specimens. Cancer cells observed in sputum are cells that are naturally exfoliated from the surface of the tumor; therefore, many of them show the final form of differentiation of the tumor or are highly degenerated dead cells. As a result, it is relatively easy to make a diagnosis of benign or malignant disease and also to determine the histologic type when such cells are present. On the other hand, in fresh cytology specimens from cases other than those accompanied by central necrosis, the cells obtained by needle cytology technique generally show no degeneration. While brushing cytology specimens contain cells with some degree of degeneration, in general most cells exhibit a low degree of degeneration. On occasion, therefore, such fresh specimens contain many immature cells or cells in the process of differentiation. As a result, even in cases of different histologic types, such as squamous cell carcinoma, adenocarcinoma or large-cell carcinoma, the morphologic appearance of cells in fresh specimens can be quite similar, thus rendering the diagnosis more difficult than that made on the basis of sputum cytology specimens. Morphologically, fresh specimen cells and nuclei tend to be large and the cytoplasm stains light green. The nuclei are round or oval, the nuclear membrance is thin and the nuclear chromatin is usually either finely granular or finely reticular.

This chapter concentrates on the morphologic appearance of fresh cytologic specimens and will also compare cells in such specimens to degenerated cancer cells observed in sputum specimens.

Even though almost all primary lung cancers originate in the epithelium of the bronchial mucosa, the histologic range of this tumor is extremely wide. Histologic types that derive from basal cells or intermediate cells of the relatively large bronchi include squamous cell carcinoma, large cell carcinoma, small cell carcinoma and adenocarcinoma (Marchesani, 1924; Okada, 1972). Adenocarcinoma, adenoid cystic carcinoma (Spencer, 1977), and mucoepidermoid carcinoma (Heilbrunn and Crosby, 1972) derive from the mucous cells and duct epithelial cells and bronchial glands, and the oat cell type of small cell carcinoma and carcinoid derive from Kulchitsky cells (Bensch, 1972). The columnar cells of the peripheral bronchi, Clara cells (Cutz and Conen, 1971; Jacques and Currie, 1977), give rise to adenocarcinoma and bronchioloalveolar carcinoma, while some alveolar cell carcinomas are still thought to derive from type-II alveolar epithelial cells of the alveolar sac, although this has not been completely established.

Table 16 Histological Classification of Lung Tumors (from the World Health Organization, 1981)

I. EPITHELIAL TUMOURS
 A. Benign
  1. Papillomas
   a. Squamous cell papilloma
   b. "Transitional" papilloma
  2. Adenomas
   a. Pleomorphic adenoma ("mixed" tumour)
   b. Monomorphic adenoma
   c. Others
 B. Dysplasia
  Carcinoma in situ
 C. Malignant
  1. Squamous cell carcinoma (epidermoid carcinoma)
   Variant:
   a. Spindle cell (squamous) carcinoma
  2. Small cell carcinoma
   a. Oat cell carcinoma
   b. Intermediate cell type
   c. Combined oat cell carcinoma
  3. Adenocarcinoma
   a. Acinar adenocarcinoma
   b. Papillary adenocarcinoma
   c. Bronchiolo-alveolar carcinoma
   d. Solid carcinoma with mucus formation
  4. Large cell carcinoma
   Variants:
   a. Giant cell carcinoma
   b. Clear cell carcinoma
  5. Adenosquamous carcinoma
  6. Carcinoid tumour
  7. Bronchial gland carcinomas
   a. Adenoid cystic carcinoma
   b. Mucoepidermoid carcinoma
   c. Others
  8. Others

II. SOFT TISSUE TUMOURS

III. MESOTHELIAL TUMOURS
 A. Benign Mesothelioma
 B. Malignant Mesothelioma
  1. Epithelial   3. Biphasic
  2. Fibrous (spindle-cell)

IV. MISCELLANEOUS TUMOURS
 A. Benign
 B. Malignant
  1. Carcinosarcoma   4. Malignant lymphomas
  2. Pulmonary blastoma 5. Others
  3. Malignant melanoma

V. SECONDARY TUMOURS

VI. UNCLASSIFIED TUMOURS

VII. TUMOUR-LIKE LESIONS
 A. Hamartoma
 B. Lymphoproliferative Lesions
 C. Tumourlet
 D. Eosinophilic Granuloma
 E. "Sclerosing Haemangioma"
 F. Inflammatory Pseudotumour
 G. Others

A classification of histologic type is necessary from the point of view of clinical treatment. The reasons for the need for a classification from the latter point of view are 1) that the natural history of the disease and the prognosis varies, depending on the histologic type and 2) that selection of therapeutic modalities is influenced by the histologic type because different types show different responses to radiotherapy and chemotherapy. For these reasons, it is important not only to be able to make a diagnosis of malignant or benign disease on the basis of cytologic criteria but also to be able to make an attempt at histologic classification.

A variety of histologic classifications have been established, including those of the World Health Organization (WHO, 1981) (Table 16). The cytologic classification used by the authors, which is a modification of the WHO histologic classification and is based primarily on the degree of differentiation, is shown in Table 17. Of these histologic types, squamous cell carcinoma, adenocarcinoma, and small cell carcinoma constitute more than 80% of all cases, as is shown in Table 18, with most of these cases being squamous cell carcinoma and adenocarcinoma.

Table 17 Cytological Classification of Lung Cancer Used in this Series

Squamous cell carcinoma
    Well differentiated
    Poorly differentiated
Small cell carcinoma
    Oat cell type
    Intermediate cell type
Adenocarcinoma
    Well differentiated
    Pooly differentiated
    Bronchioloalveolar type
Large cell carcinoma
    Giant cell type
Adenosquamous Carcinoma
Carcinoid
Adenoid cystic carcinoma
Mucoepidermoid carcinoma
Carcinosarcoma
Others

Table 18 Breakdown of Lung Cancer According to Histologic Type

Author	Year	No. of cases	Squamous cell ca.	Adenoca.	Small cell ca.	Large cell ca.	Others
Vincent	1977	1682	38.0%	26.5%	19.2%	9.3%	6.9%
Cox	1979	1017	33.0%	28.2%	22.1%		16.6%
Suemasu	1978	656	32.9%	41.8%	12.7%		12.6%
Hayata	1980	1441	40.8%	39.8%	8.7%	9.6%	1.3%

SQUAMOUS CELL CARCINOMA

Squamous cell carcinoma is the most common histologic type of lung cancer. It shows a tendency to originate in large bronchi and has been associated with a variety of reported carcinogens, such as tobacco smoke and air pollution. The tendency toward cellular degeneration is strong. Squamous cell carcinoma tends to invade along the bronchial wall and be exposed in the bronchial lumen. Cavity formation is frequently recognized.

The authors subdivided this histologic type into well differentiated squamous cell carcinoma in which keratinizing cells are commonly observed (Fig. 93), and poorly differentiated squamous cell carcinoma in which almost no keratinizing cells can be recognized (Fig. 94). The more distal the site of origin of a squamous cell carcinoma, the greater the likelihood that it is poorly differentiated.

Clinical Findings: (X-ray film) Since squamous cell carcinoma has a tendency to develop in larger bronchi, X-ray findings frequently show a shadow in the hilar region and as this histologic type frequently grows replacing the ciliated epithelium, the cilia transport mechanism is disturbed. This can cause accumulation of mucus which appears on X-ray as secondary changes or atelectasis. If squamous cell carcinoma develops in the periphery of the lung, it frequently shows cavity formation. In cases of early stage squamous cell carcinoma, the X-ray film generally shows no abnormalities.
(Fiberoptic Bronchoscopy) A white necrotic substance on the surface of the tumor is a characteristic finding in the case of well differentiated squamous cell carcinoma. On the contrary, no necrotic substance is observed in poorly differentiated squamous cell carcinoma.

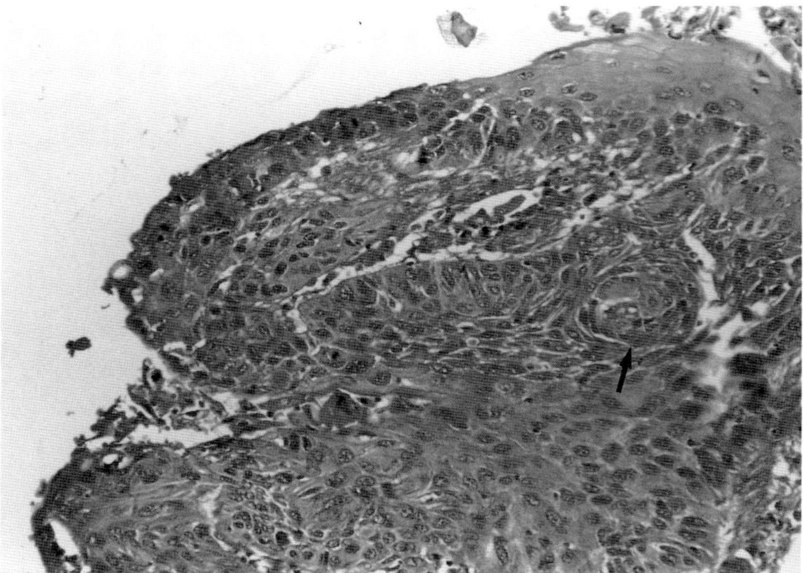

Fig. 93 Well differentiated squamous cell carcinoma. Histologically keratinization is prominent throughout the whole layer of squamous cell carcinoma. Cancer pearls can be seen (arrows).
(X100, H.E.)

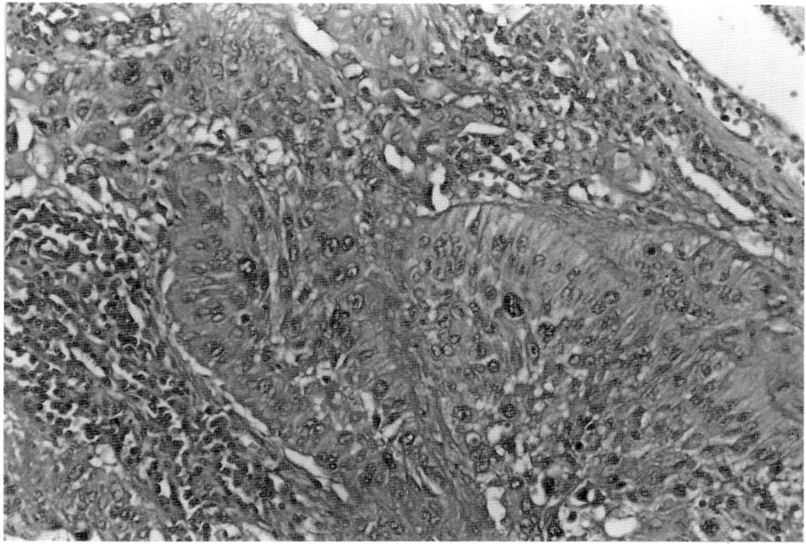

Fig. 94 Poorly differentiated squamous cell carcinoma. Keratinization and intracellular bridges are absent in this histologic specimen. Solid nests with fascicular arrangement and a moderate amount of eosinophilic cytoplasm indicate squamous differentiation. (X200, H.E.)

Well Differentiated

Sputum cytology specimens

Most well differentiated squamous cell carcinoma cells observed in sputum specimens possess cytoplasm that stains with Orange G, as shown in Figure 95a. Keratinized cancer cells often appear as single cells. Morphologically, the cells are bizarre and show a variety of appearances (Figs. 96–99). The dense, amorphous nuclei stain homogeneously, nucleoli are usually not recognizable and necrotic substances are frequently observed in the background.

Brushing and needle cytology specimens

Due to the nature of the specimen harvesting method, brushing and curettage specimens contain clusters of cells more frequently than do sputum specimens, and the appearance of keratinized squamous cell carcinoma cells is less frequent. The brushing cytology specimen, obtained from the same case as that illustrated in Figures 93 and 95a, is shown in Figures 95b, c. The cells are slightly larger, the cytoplasm stains basophilic and many nonkeratinized squamous cell carcinoma cells can be seen. The cytoplasm in general is thickened, with a concentric circular pattern, and stains eosinophilic in part (Fig. 100). These findings indicate that it is in the process of differentiation to a keratinized state. The nuclei are located in the center of the cells but show wide variation in form and size. The nuclear membrane is thin but not smooth. The chromatin is finely granular to reticular. Several prominent nucleoli can usually be observed but their shapes are irregular. When the cells appear in clusters, they point in one direction; when they appear in sheets, their arrangement resembles that of cobblestones.

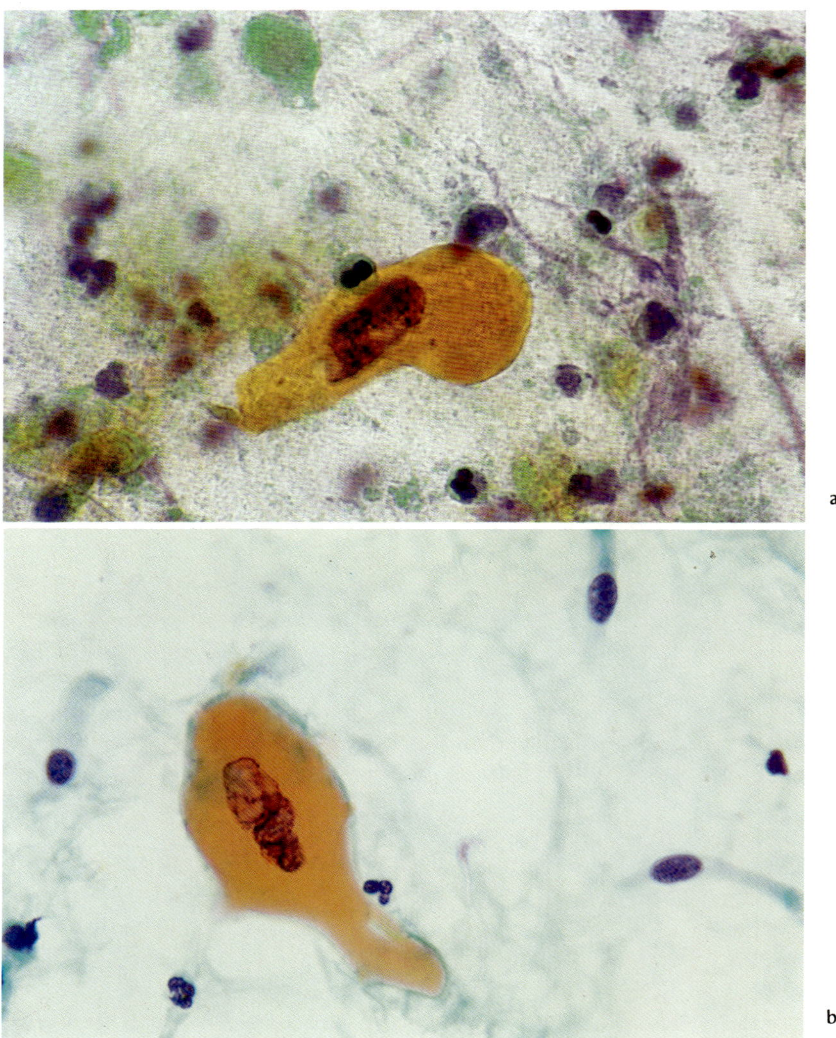

Fig. 95 See legend on opposite page.

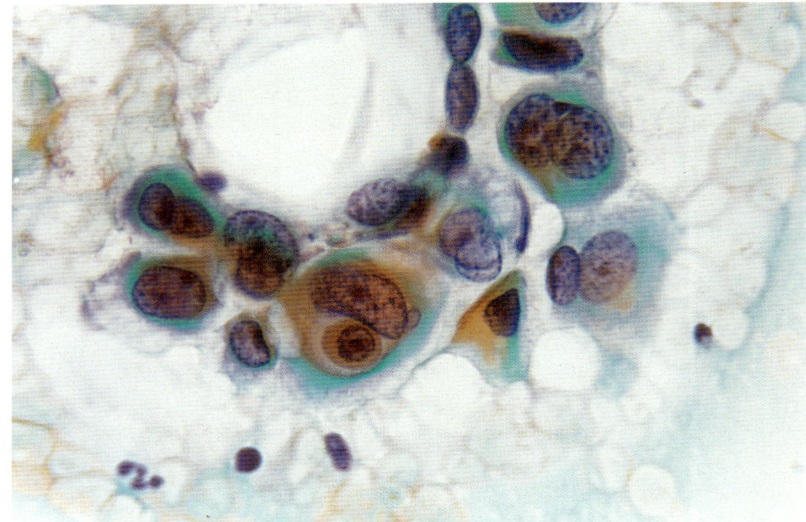

c

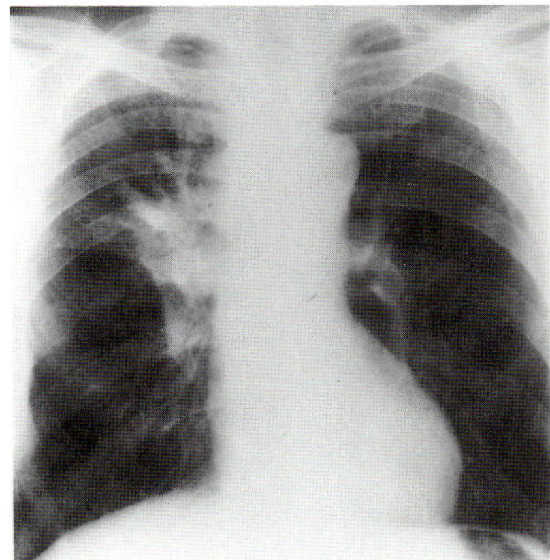

d

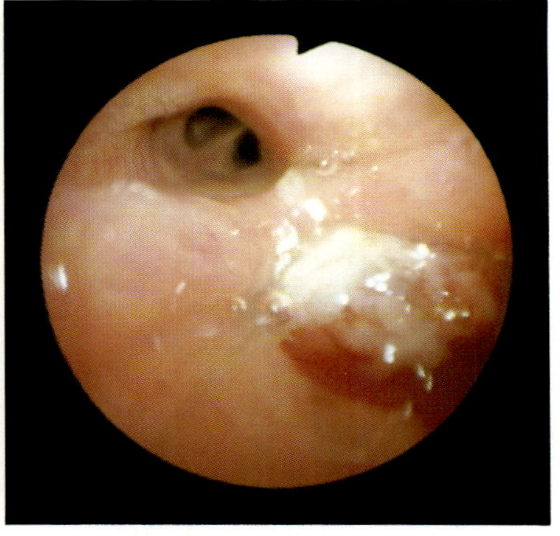

e

Fig. 95 Keratinizing squamous cell carcinoma in the case shown in Figure 93.

(a) Sputum cytology specimen. The nucleus of the bizarrely-shaped cell stains darkly. The intranuclear structure cannot be recognized but the cytoplasm is brightly orangeophilic. Hyperchromasia is prominent and nucleoli are not clearly recognizable. Necrotic materials can be seen in the background. Well differentiated squamous cell carcinoma. (X400, Pap.)

(b) Transbroncial brushing cytology specimen showing a well differentiated squamous cell carcinoma cell. The cytoplasm stains eosinophilically. The nuclear shape is irregular and the nuclear chromatin is granular with clumps of chromatin around the nuclear border. (X400, Pap.)

(c) Another group of cancer cells in a transbronchial brushing cytology specimen with clusters of cells showing relatively little adhesion. The cytoplasm stains basophilically. The nuclei are polygonal, the chromatin is finely granular and small irregular nucleoli are recognized. The same cells show keratinization. (X400, Pap.)

(d) The chest X-ray film shows an infiltrative shadow in the right hilar region. This shadow indicates the obstruction of a large bronchus. Squamous cell carcinoma frequently develops in the larger bronchis.

(e) Fiberoptic bronchoscopic findings of well differentiated squamous cell carcinoma in the right upper lobe bronchus. This bronchus is obstructed completely with necrotic material, which is one of the characteristic findings of this type of carcinoma.

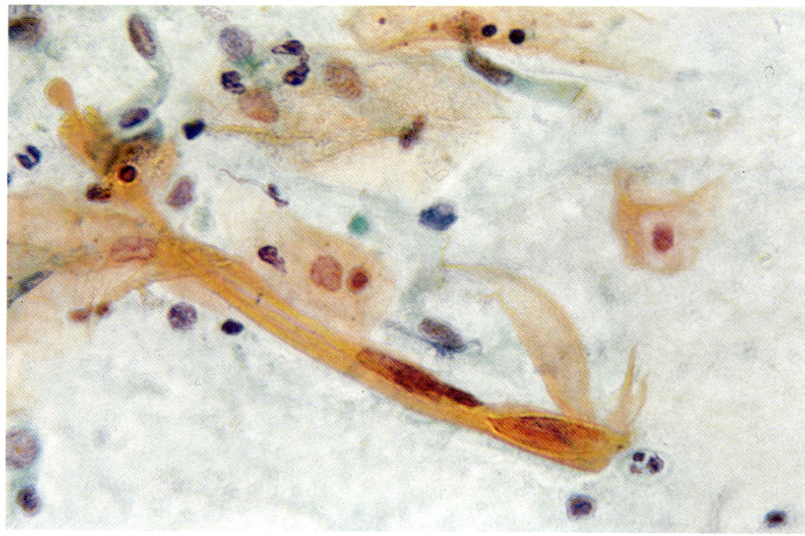

Fig. 96 Well differentiated squamous cell carcinoma in a sputum cytology specimen. Exfoliated spindle-like cell with keratinizing cytoplasm indicates this type of carcinoma. The nucleus shows hyperchromasia. (X400, Pap.)

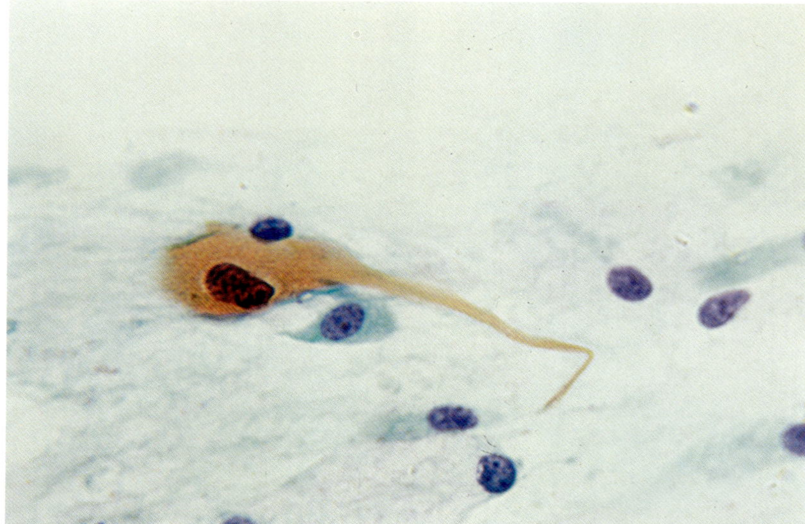

Fig. 97 Well differentiated squamous cell carcinoma in a sputum cytology specimen. In a bizarre cell with a keratinizing long tail, the nucleus shows hyperchromasia with coarse chromatin. (X400, Pap.)

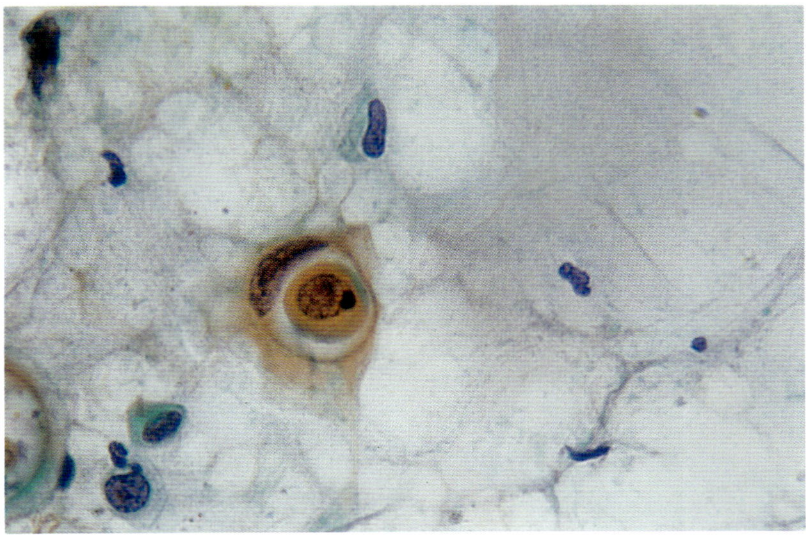

Fig. 98 Well differentiated squamous cell carcinoma in a sputum cytology specimen. Cannibalism and keratinizing cytoplasm indicate well differentiated squamous cell carcinoma. (X400, Pap.)

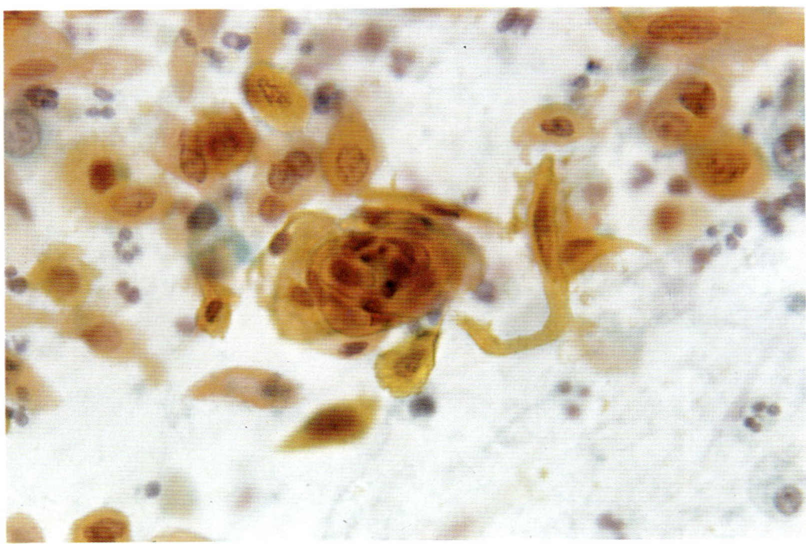

Fig. 99 Well differentiated squamous cell carcinoma in a sputum cytology specimen. Cancer pearls with keratinizing cytoplasm and hyperchromatic nuclei are characteristic. (X400, Pap.)

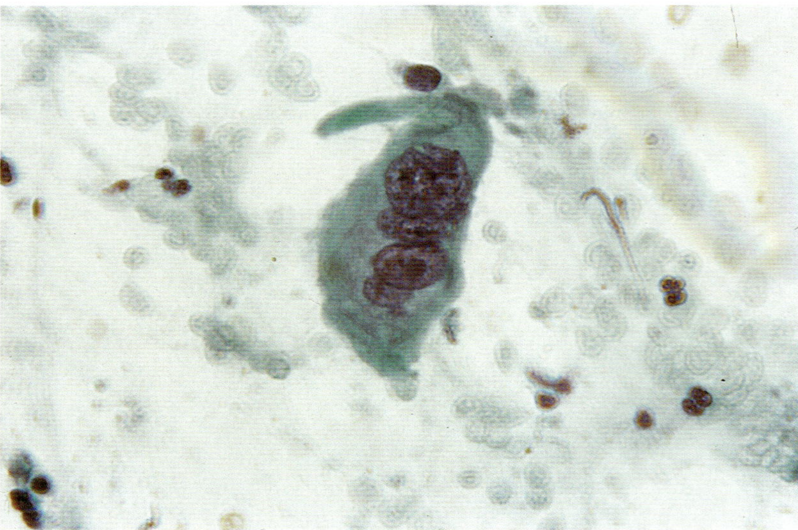

Fig. 100 Well differentiated squamous cell carcinoma in a brushing cytology specimen. Multinucleic large cells with basophilic cytoplasm are frequently seen in brushing cytology specimens in cases of well differentiated squamous cell carcinoma. Thickened cytoplasm and hyperchromatic nucleus indicate squamous cell carcinoma. (X400, Pap.)

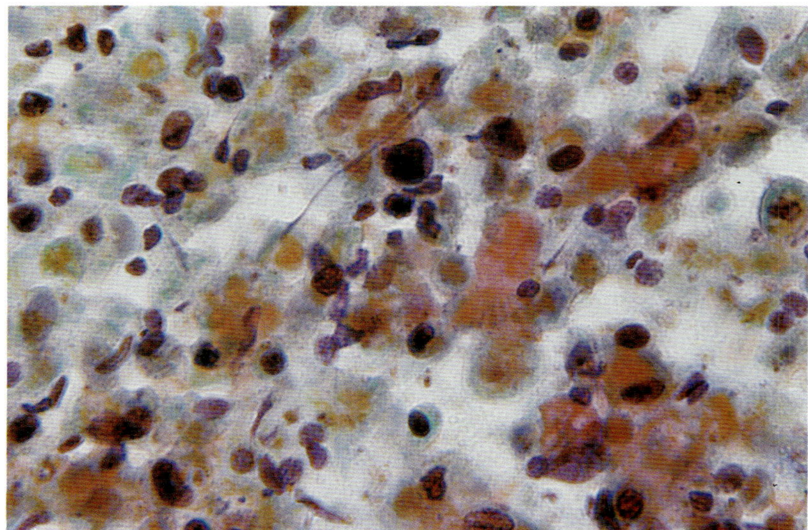

Fig. 101 Well differentiated squamous cell carcinoma in a needle aspiration cytology specimen. This specimen was obtained from the center of the lesion. Squamous cell carcinoma frequently shows necrosis in the center of the focus, therefore necrosis, ghost cells and keratinizing squamous cell carcinoma cells can be seen. (X400, Pap.)

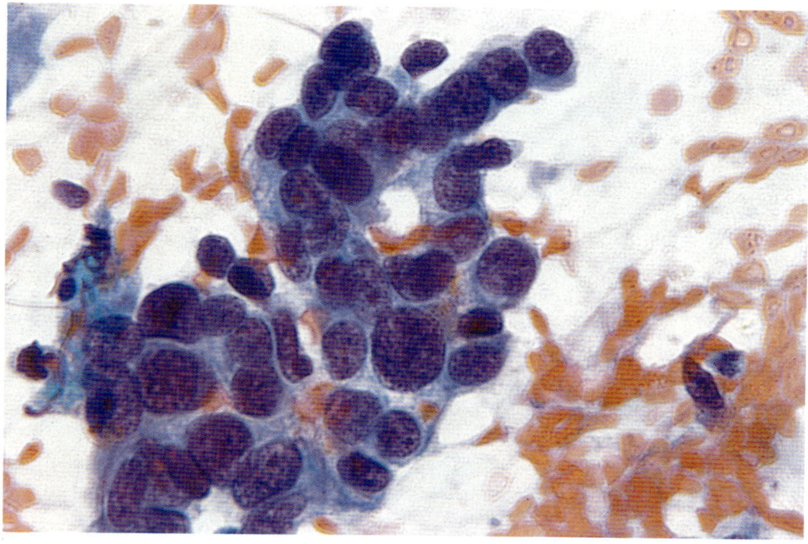

Fig. 102 Well differentiated squamous cell carcinoma in a needle aspiration cytology specimen. This specimen was obtained from the margin of the lesion. These cells are less differentiated and may be thought of as tumor stem cells. Hyperchromatic nuclei indicate squamous cell carcinoma. The cytoplasm is scanty, frothy and stains basophilically. (X400, Pap.)

The greater the degree of differentiation of squamous cell carcinoma, the greater the tendency for the development of necrosis at the center of the lesion. As a result, needle cytology specimens obtained from the center of the lesion tend to show characteristics of degeneration and necrosis (Fig. 101). Cells from the tumor margin, however, show poorly differentiated, non-necrotic cells with little degeneration (Fig. 102).

As described above, a relatively large number of keratinized squamous cell carcinoma cells can be observed in brushing/curettage and needle cytology specimens, thereby rendering the diagnosis of squamous cell carcinoma relatively simple.

Poorly Differentiated

Sputum cytology specimens

Poorly differentiated squamous cell carcinoma cells seen in sputum specimens do not exhibit the orange G stainability observed in well differentiated squamous cell carcinoma cells, and most of the cells observed are poorly differentiated cells that stain basophilic. The appearance of clusters or sheets of cells is rare, the most frequent appearance being as single cells. Since the cells have been exfoliated, they display a high degree of degeneration, with occasional degenerated vacuoles recognizable in the cytoplasm. The nuclear chromatin appears as aggregated clumps or pyknotic lumps; therefore, the appearance is coarsely granular to coarsely reticular. The nuclear border is irregular. The diagnosis of squamous cell carcinoma can be made on the basis of thickened cytoplasm, the eosinophilic staining of parts of a small number of cells, hyperchromasia and the irregularity of the nuclear border (Fig. 103a).

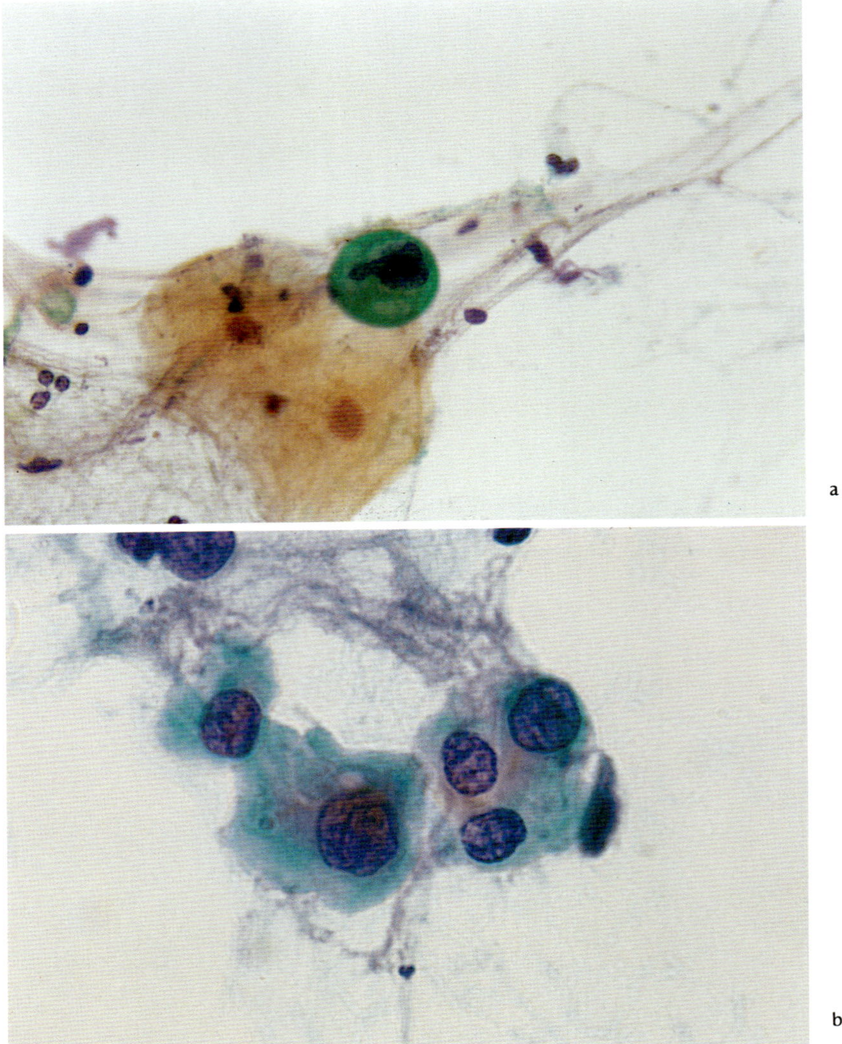

Fig. 103 Poorly differentiated squamous cell carcinoma of the case shown in Figure 94.
(a) Sputum cytology specimen. The thickened cytoplasm stains basophilically. The nuclear chromatin is coarsely granular and irregularity of the nuclear membrane is recognized. A halo is seen around the nucleus. These findings suggest squamous cell carcinoma. (X400, Pap.)
(b) Brushing cytology specimen. Coarse chromatin and clumping at the irregular nuclear membrane are seen. Hyperchromasia is not prominent but thickened basophilic cytoplasm suggests poorly differentiated squamous cell carcinoma. (X400, Pap.)

Brushing and needle cytology specimens

Brushing and needle cytology specimens of poorly differentiated squamous cell carcinoma exhibit a low degree of degeneration, the cytoplasm stains frothily basophilic and there are few degenerative vacuoles (Fig. 104). Sometimes, the cell borders are unclear and the cytoplasm is scanty (Fig. 103b). The nuclei possess thin borders and have finely reticular chromatin, while the prominent nucleoli show irregularity (Fig. 105). It is extremely difficult to differentiate these features from those of large cell carcinoma or poorly differentiated adeno-carcinoma. However, it is usually possible to make a correct diagnosis of poorly differentiated squamous cell carcinoma by scanning the entire specimen to detect a certain tendency to keratinize in the cytoplasm of some cells (Fig. 106). Other features that can be used to diagnose squamous cell carcinoma definitively include sheets of cells presenting a cobblestone-like appearance, clumps of chromatin along the nuclear borders and the frequency of irregular nuclear borders and irregular nucleoli.

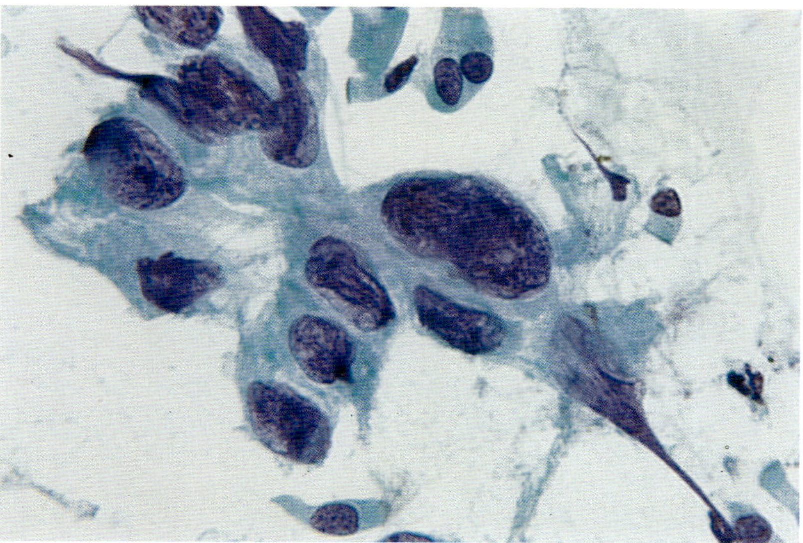

Fig. 104 Poorly differentiated squamous cell carcinoma in a brushing cytology specimen. Variation of nuclear size, striking hyperchromasia are prominent findings in this specimen. Cytoplasm stains frothily basophilic. Nucleic findings only suggest squamous cell carcinoma. (X400, Pap.)

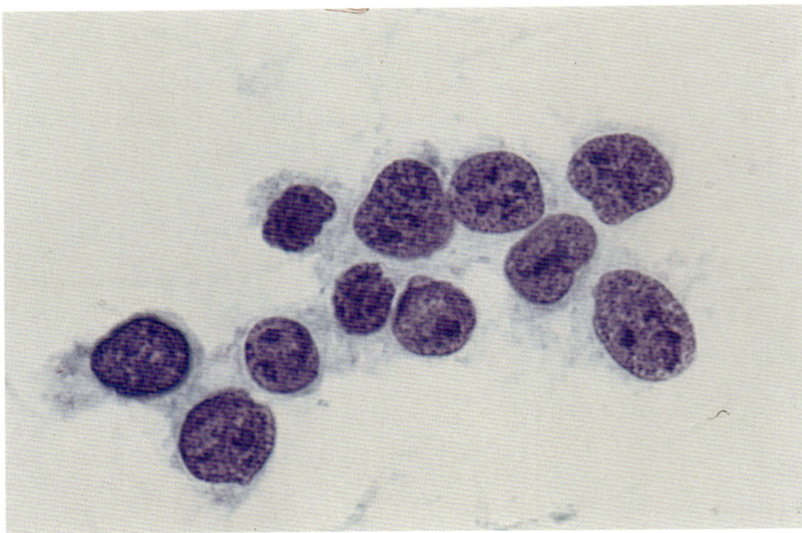

Fig. 105 Poorly differentiated squamous cell carcinoma in a needle cytology specimen. Chromatin is granular and multiple nucleoli are seen. Nuclear membrane is thin and some nuclei show hyperchromasia. Cytoplasm is frothy but scanty. It is sometimes difficult to make a differential diagnosis of squamous cell carcinoma or adenocarcinoma in such poorly differentiated carcinoma cases. (X400, Pap.)

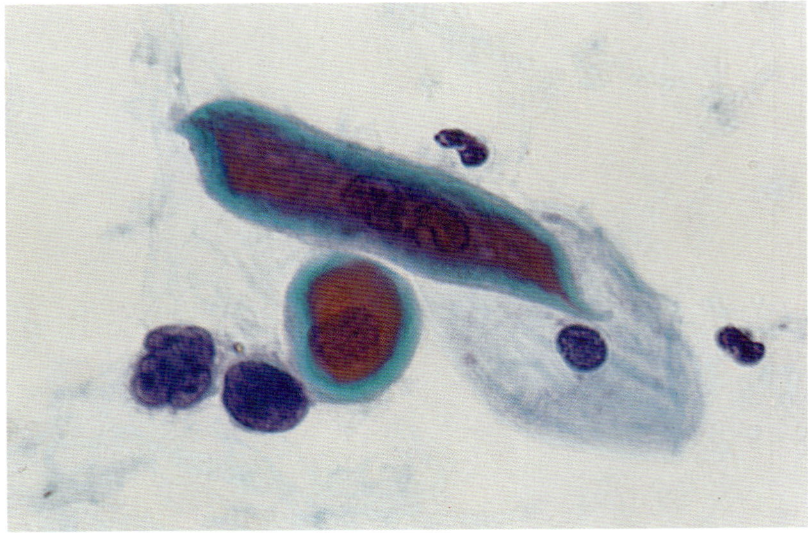

Fig. 106 Poorly differentiated squamous cell carcinoma in a brushing cytology specimen. Tendency for cytoplasm to keratinize is a help to make a diagnosis of squamous cell carcinoma in cases of poorly differentiated carcinoma. (X400, Pap.)

In Situ Carcinoma

Carcinoma in situ or intraepithelial carcinoma is a histologic term signifying a squamous cell carcinoma limited to within the bronchial epithelium without breaking through the basement membrane (Fig. 107c, d). It is difficult to diagnose carcinoma in situ on the basis of cytologic findings alone. A definitive diagnosis requires endoscopic and histologic examination. However some characteristic features can be depicted as described below. Histologic criteria have been defined by Black and Ackerman (1952).

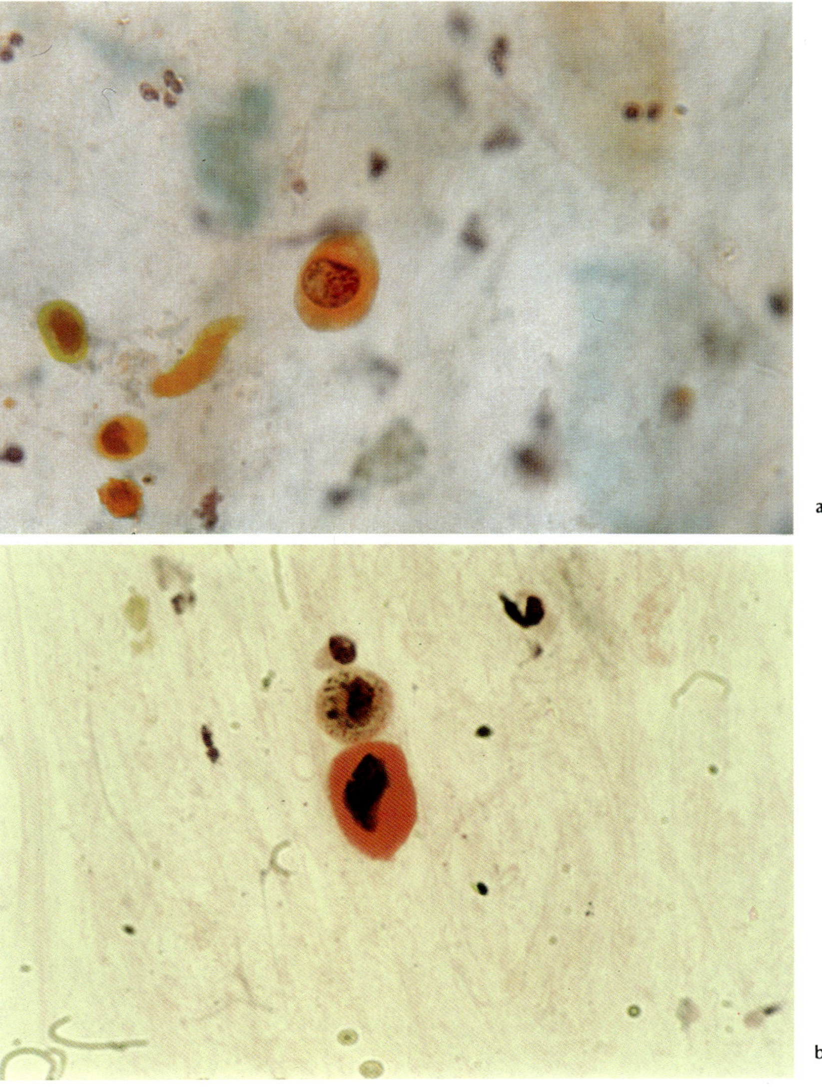

Fig. 107   See legend on page 90.

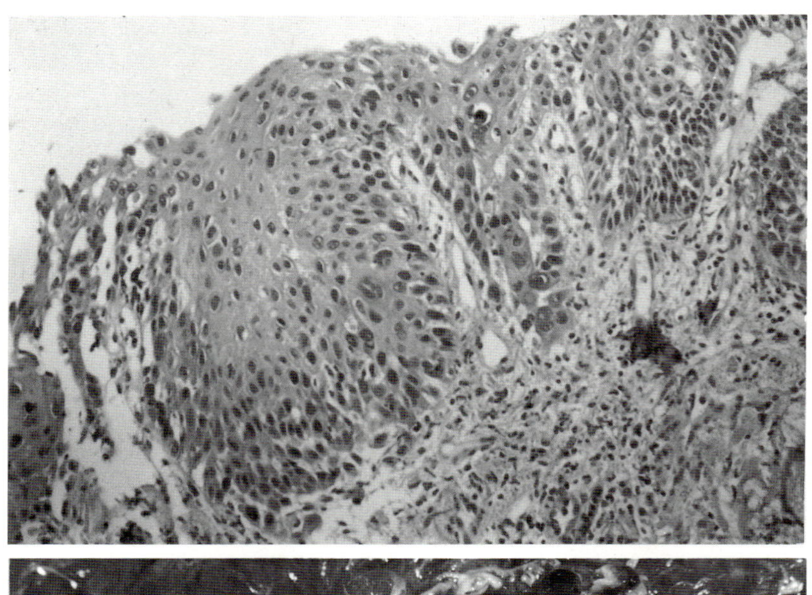

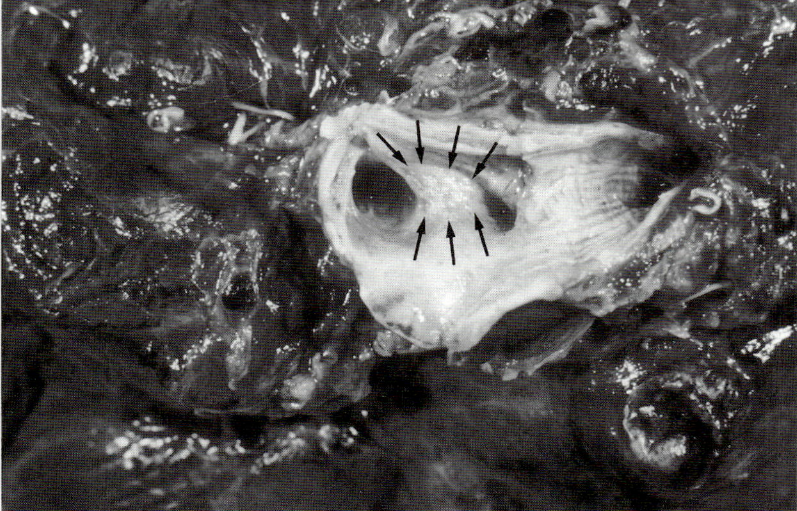

Fig. 107 Carcinoma in situ.

(a) Sputum cytology specimen. Chromatin is coarsely granular and clumped at the nuclear membrane. The cytoplasm shows keratinization. These findings yielded a diagnosis of carcinoma in situ. The small single cell, oval in shape is characteristic. (X400, Pap.)

(b) Brushing cytology specimen. Small cancer cells are seen. Most carcinoma in situ cells are smaller than those of invasive carcinoma. Nuclear hyperchromasia is not prominent. Nucleoli are seen and cytoplasm shows dark basophilic staining. The background appears clean. (X400, Pap.)

(c) Histology of surgical specimen. The proliferation of the carcinoma cells is limited to the mucosal epithelium, and the basement membrane can be observed to be preserved. The cellular arrangement is irregular and mitosis can be seen. Squamous metaplasia is seen adjacent to carcinoma in situ. (X200, H.E.)

(d) Surgical specimen. The lesion of the case shows only a slight degree of irregularity at the bifurcation of B^{1+2} and B^3.

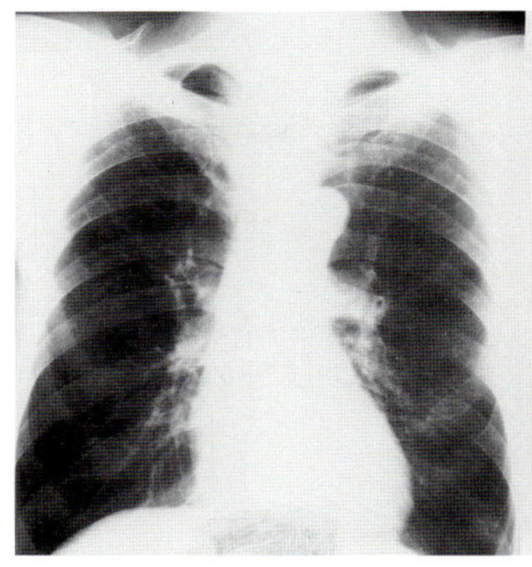

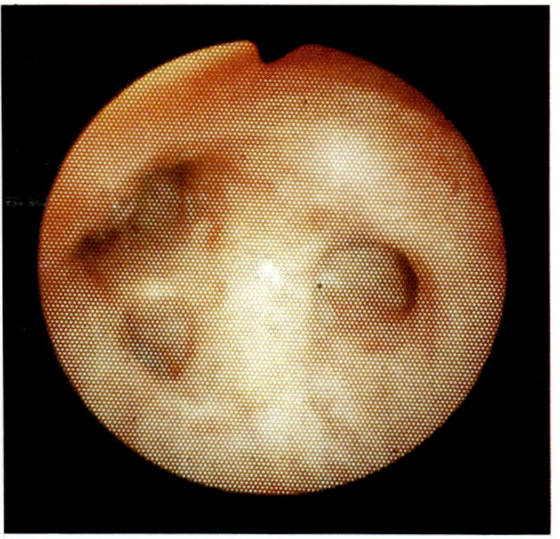

Fig. 107 (continued)
(e)   Chest X-ray film which revealed no abnormal findings. This case was a 51-year-old male heavy smoker detected in a mass survey of a residential area of Tokyo.
(f)   Fiberoptic bronchoscopic findings. Slightly irregular mucosa at the bifurcation of left B^{1+2} and B^3 was recognized by fiberoptic bronchoscopy. While in some cases of carcinoma in situ no irregularity whatsoever can be recognized by fiberoptic bronchoscopy, the most common endoscopic findings are thickening of the mucosal membrane, reddening, loss of the gloss of the mucosal membrane and irregularity.

Clinical Findings: (Chest X-ray) No abnormal findings are observed in the chest X-ray film (Fig. 107e).
(Fiberoptic Bronchoscopy) Carcinoma in situ can appear as mucosal thickening, irregularly and redness, but some cases exhibit no endoscopic abnormality (Fig. 107f).

Sputum cytology specimens

The cytologic characteristics of carcinoma in situ cells in sputum specimens have been described by Woolner (1973), Nasiell (1979) (Table 19) and Saccomanno (1978) (Table 20) as relatively small cells with a clean background, but cytologists now encounter ever-increasing amounts of fresh cells that have been obtained directly from the lesion due to important developments in fiberoptic broncho-scopic techniques (Kato and Konaka, 1982).

Carcinoma in situ cells appear as small single cells (cells greater than 300 μm^2 in size are rare), round or oval in shape (Figs. 107a and 108). The cytoplasm is organgeophilic and the nucleic structure shows the same characteristics as

Table 19   Abnormal Cells from in situ Carcinoma.
(from Nasiell, M.: Compendium on Diagnostic Cytology, 4th ed., Tutorials of Cytology, Chicago, 1979. pp. 315—329)

1.   Carcinoma cells which fulfill the requirements for epidermoid carcinoma, possibly less bizarre in appearance than those of classical invasive type.

2.   Small abnormal squamous cells usually round to oval and showing evidence of cell keratinization.

3.   Large cells, polygonal, round or irregular in shape with abundant usually orange-ophilic, or eosinophilic cytoplasm and enlarged, slightly hyperchromatic nuclei.

The occurrence of many *single* abnormal cells and a *"clean"* background are other characteristics of in situ or early infiltrative epidermoid carcinoma of the lung.

Table 20 Carcinoma in situ. (from Saccomanno, G.: Diagnostic Pulmonary Cytology, American Society of Clinical Pathologists, Chicago, 1978)

1. Cells vary in size and may be double the size of marked metaplasia. Single cells are present, but clusters are more common than in invasive carcinoma.

2. The nuclear material is coarse and accumulates in large masses, but the concentrations are not usually accumulated near the membrane. Chromocenters are large and simulate nucleoli, but are not always acidophilic.

3. The nuclear/cytoplasmic ratio is decreased in some, while increased in others, causing obvious nuclear pleomorphism.

4. Cannibalism and multinucleation may be present.

5. Acidophilic cytoplasm predominates.

invasive squamous cell carcinoma cells. A clean background is a characteristic finding because they are not accompanied by tumor diathesis. Occasionally large cells are observed.

Brushing cytology specimens

Fresh cells differ in some respects from cells exfoliated from tumors that are found in sputum specimens. The criteria established by the authors for diagnosing carcinoma in situ in fresh specimens are shown in Table 21.

The cells are usually obtained in clusters. Cellular adhesion is relatively noticeable, and in this respect these cells closely resemble those of severely atypical squamous metaplasia. However the number of abnormal cells is greater than in squamous metaplasia. Single cells are sometimes observed, and there is little variation in cellular size. Since single cells in specimens generally derive from the superficial stratum, the cytoplasm shows a strong tendency toward keratinization,

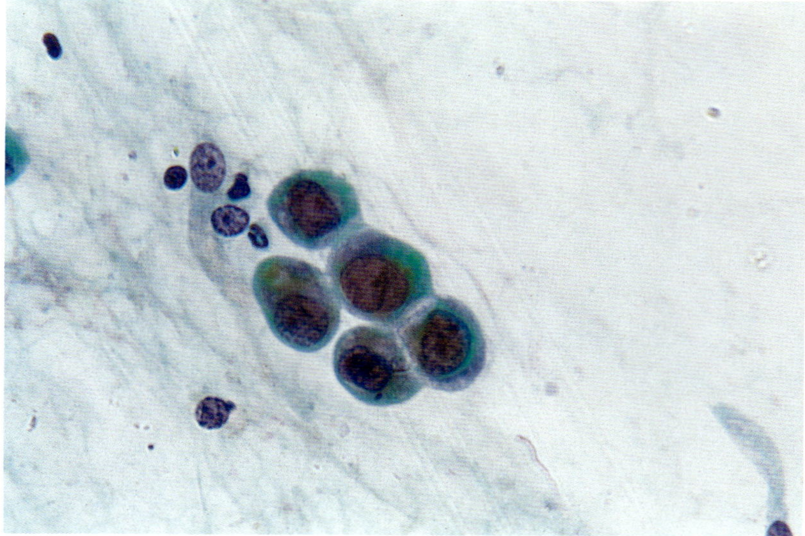

Fig. 108 Carcinoma in situ in a sputum cytology specimen. The cytoplasm of a single small round cell stains orange and displays keratinization. The round nucleus is strikingly chromatic; the chromatin is coarsely granular and the nuclear membrane is irregular. The background is clean. (X400, Pap.)

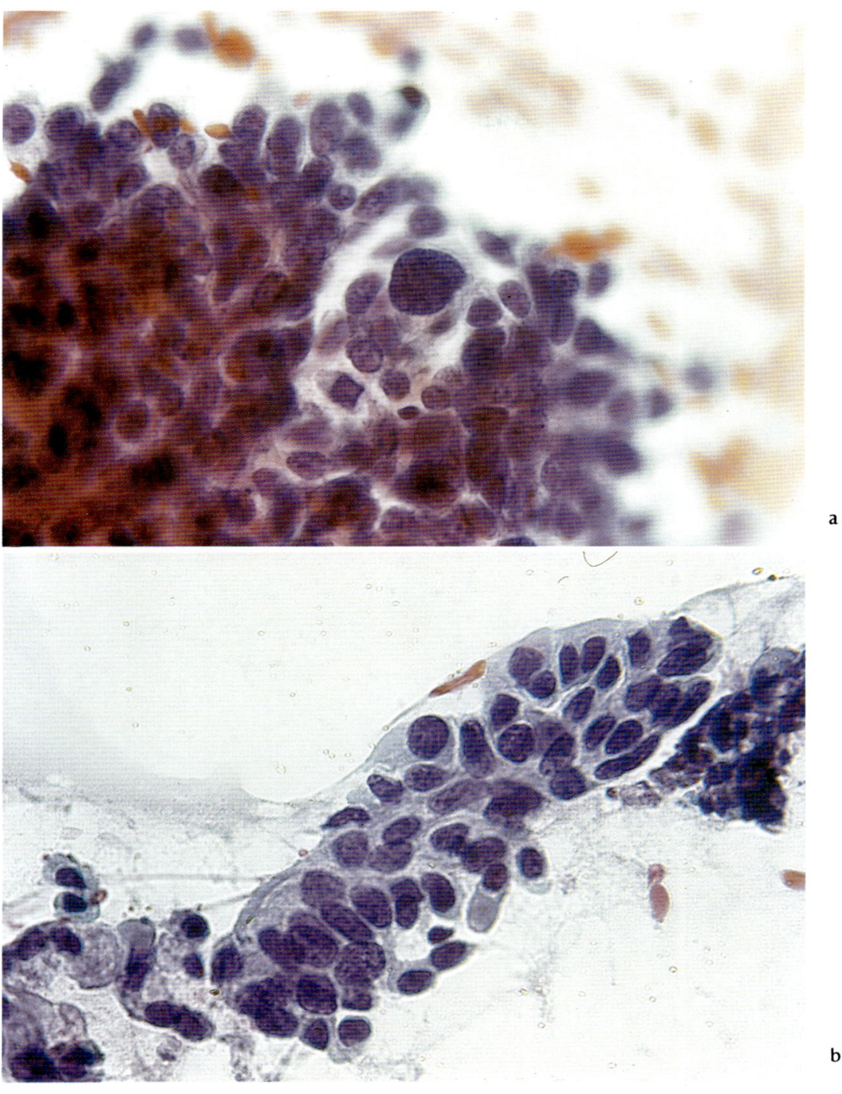

Fig. 109 Carcinoma in situ.
(a)   Brushing cytology specimen. Cells are obtained frequently as clusters by brushing cells in the center show strong hyperchromasia and most cells in this specimen suggest carcinoma in situ. (X400, Pap.)
(b)   Brushing cytology specimen. Hyperchromasia is a characteristic finding in this specimen. The finely granular chromatin is due to the very limited degeneration in comparison to the sputum cytology specimen. (X400, Pap.)

staining orange. On the other hand, clusters usually contain cells from layers below the surface; therefore, the cytoplasm frequently stains light green.

Single cells are usually small (300 μm^2 or less) and are typically round or oval. The size of the nucleus is less than 120 μm^2. Large cells, appearing in a variety of shapes are occasionally recognized, but in such cases there is not an intense increase in the amount of nuclear chromatin.

The chromatin is usually granular. The nucleoli are irregular, with usually one or more per cell. Although the nucleoli can be large, they are sometimes hidden

Table 21 Cytomorphology of Carcinoma in situ in Brushing Specimens

1. Cells still occur in clusters. Cellular arrangement is pavement-like with striking overlapping. Single cells are more frequent in the cluster than in severely atypical metaplasia.
2. Cytoplasms of cluster cells stain light green but single cells display eosinophilic tendencies.
3. Nuclear shape is variable.
4. Nuclear membrane is irregular.
5. Chromatin is granular sometimes coarsely, and hyperchromasia is distinct.
6. Nucleoli are irregular.
7. The nuclear to cytoplasmic ratio is large.
8. The background to the cells is clean.

by abundant chromatin (Figs. 107b and 109a, b).

The background to the cells is clean, with no necrosis due to tumor diathesis. There is no appreciable difference between carcinoma in situ and invasive carcinoma in terms of the nuclear to cytoplasmic ratio, chromatin distribution or amount of DNA.

SMALL CELL CARCINOMA

Small cell carcinoma is an undifferentiated tumor that shows the greatest degree of malignancy of all the histologic types of lung cancer. It displays a tendency to develop in large bronchi, proliferating invasively, and shows early lymphatic and hematogenous metastasis (Fig. 110d). This histologic type is divided into subtypes, oat cell carcinoma (Fig. 110c), which consists of cells that resemble lymphocytes, and intermediate cell carcinoma (Fig. 112d) which is composed of slightly larger, polygonal cells.

Clinical Findings: (Chest X-ray) Rapid lymphnode involvement is clinically characteristic, therefore hilar and mediastinal enlargements are generally observed.
(Fiberoptic Bronchoscopy) The tumor tends to extend submucosally, occasionally breaking through the bronchial mucosa. Therefore, tumor is generally observed with swelling of the mucosa.

Oat Cell Type

Sputum cytology specimens

The oat cell type of small cell carcinoma appears in sputum specimens as loose clusters of cells that exhibit a low degree of cellular adhesion, and a necrotic background is frequent. The cells are small and resemble lymphocytes. The cytoplasm is scanty and sometimes has disappeared due to degeneration during exfoliation. The nuclei are round, oval or irregular and display variation in size. Due to degeneration, the nuclear chromatin is pyknotic and frequently appears like a dot of India ink (Fig. 110a), although in cases in which there is little degeneration it may be finely granular (Fig. 111a). Some cells show small nucleoli.

Because Saccomanno's method disperses the cells, when the number of cells is small the oat cell type of small cell carcinoma is usually difficult to recognize in specimens prepared by this method, and thus cases may be overlooked on screening.

Brushing and needle cytology specimens

Specimens of the oat cell type of small cell carcinoma obtained by brushing/curettage or by the needle cytology technique show a relatively low degree of degeneration, and the cells are usually larger than those seen in sputum specimens. The cytoplasm stains basophilic, and the cellular borders are easily destroyed and unclear. The nuclear membranes are thin, the chromatin is finely to coarsely granular and several nucleoli can be recognized (Figs. 110b and 111b).

The cells can easily be destroyed by the mechanical process of obtaining and preparing specimens, and destroyed or smudged nuclei are occasionally seen. Closely overlapping clusters of cells are observed.

Intermediate Cell Type

Sputum cytology specimens

The cells of the intermediate cell type of small cell carcinoma are larger than those of the oat cell type, and the cytoplasm is often polygonal. The nuclear chromatin is also not as pyknotic as that of the oat cell type, and the intranuclear structure can be recognized. One or two nucleoli can be recognized, even in degenerated cells in sputum specimens. The cytoplasm in this type is more abundant than in the oat cell type, and the cell borders are unclear. Sheets of cells showing a low degree of cellular adhesion can be seen in sputum specimens (Fig. 112a).

Brushing and needle cytology specimens

The undegenerated cells of the intermediate cell type are larger than those seen in sputum specimens, and they show great variation in size. The cytoplasm is more abundant than in the oat cell type and is destroyed easily, and the cellular borders are unclear. The shape of the nuclei is irregular, and the nuclear borders are smooth. The chromatin is coarsely granular, and nucleoli are usually recognized.

Brushing specimens often show overlapping clusters of cells due to its technical characteristics in spite of a low degree of cellular adhesion. Cells are sometimes destroyed by the collection and preparation method. Necrotic material is frequently recognized in the background (Fig. 112b, c).

The differential diagnosis of intermediate cell type from poorly differentiated cell carcinoma and carcinoid tumor is sometimes difficult. The features of squamous cell carcinoma cells that serve to distinguish it are the abundant, thickened cytoplasm overlapping and their regular thickening of the nuclear borders. Intermediate cell type has thinner, paler cytoplasm and lacks hyperchromatism. In the case of carcinoid tumor cells, abundant, pale finely granular cytoplasm and uniformity of nuclear size and shape are the differential features from intermediate cell type of small cell carcinoma. In intermediate cell type carcinoma there is considerable variation in nuclear size.

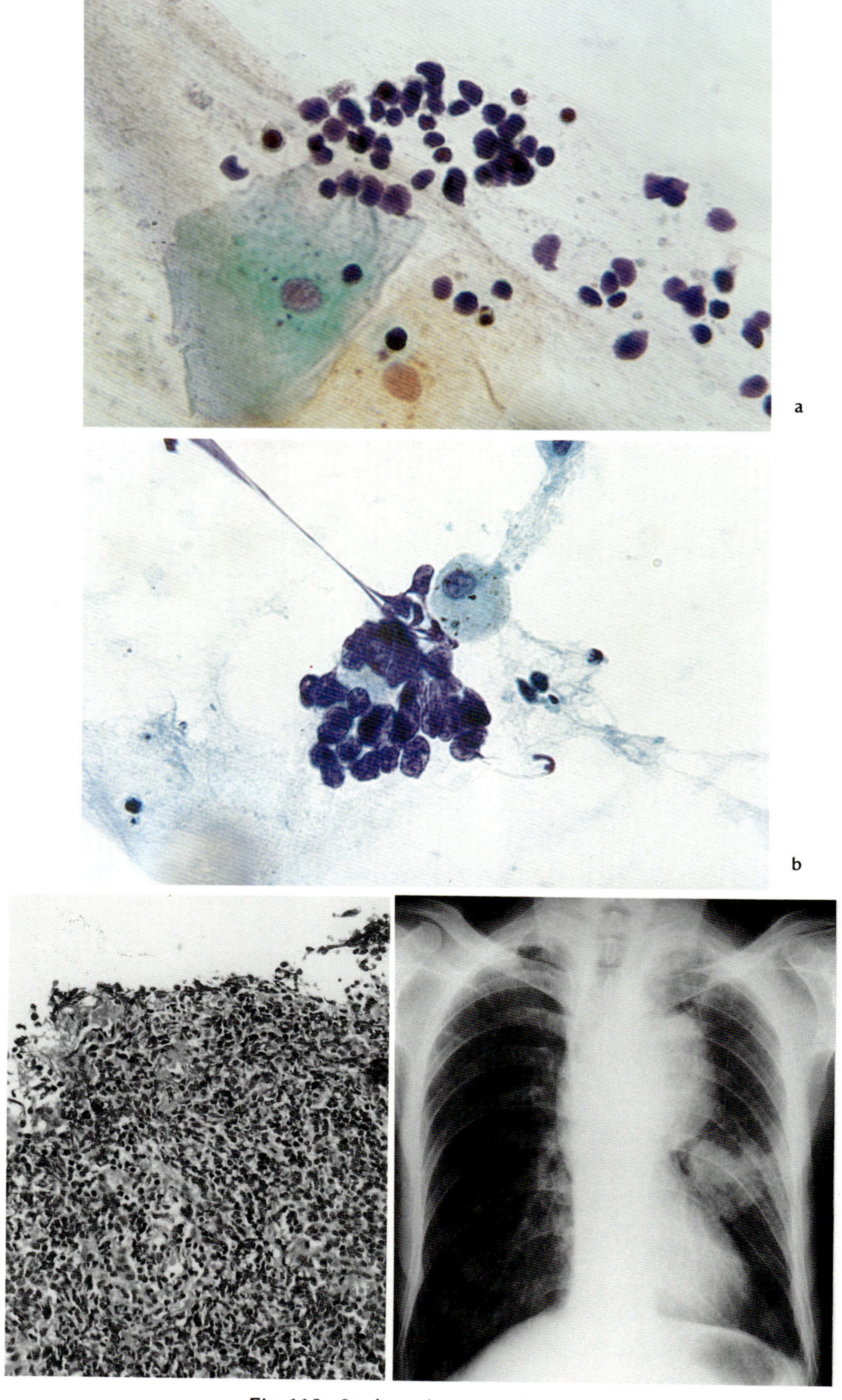

Fig. 110   See legend on opposite page.

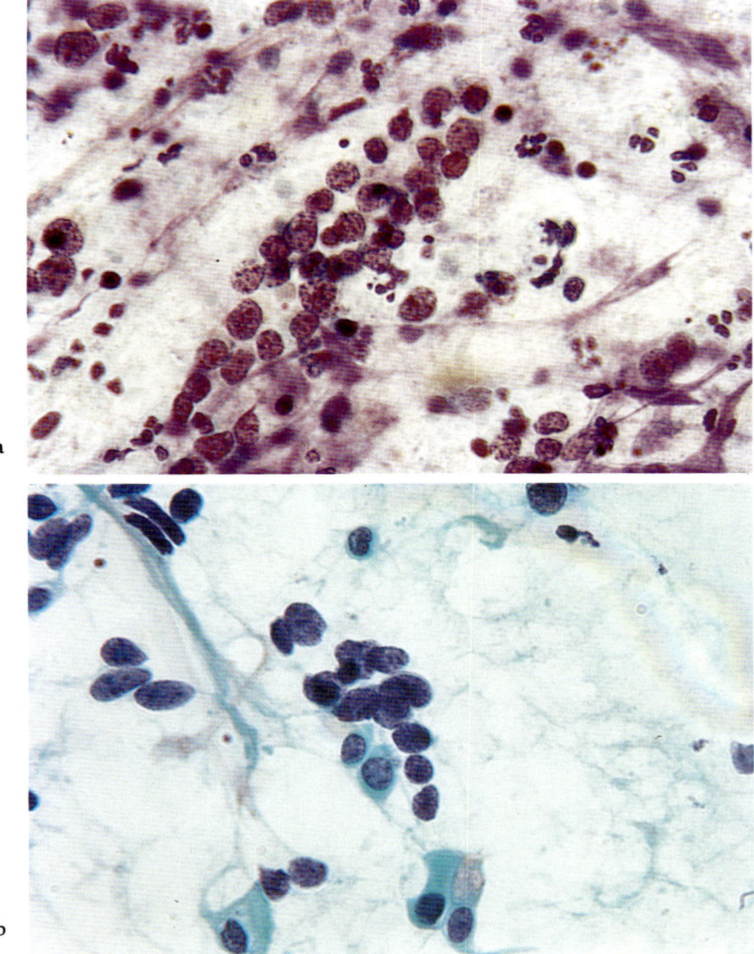

Fig. 111 Small cell carcinoma, oat cell type.
(a) Sputum cytology specimen. In sputum specimens, degenerative cells are sometimes observed as shown in this figure. Chromatin is coarse and clumped at nuclear membrane. (X400, Pap.)
(b) Brushing cytology specimen. Cells have scanty cytoplasm with unclear borders. The chromatin of the round nuclei is granular and dense, and nucleoli can be seen. The nuclei of these cells, which exhibit little degeneration, can be clearly recognized. (X400, Pap.)

Fig. 110 Small cell carcinoma, oat cell type.
(a) Sputum cytology specimen. Clusters of cells with small dense nuclei and scanty cytoplasm are seen. The chromatin is also highly hyperchromatic, resembling Indian ink. Necrosis can be recognized in the background. (X400, Pap.)
(b) Brushing cytology specimen. The adhesive cells with irregularly sized nuclei in the cluster possessing coarsely granular chromatin and nucleoli cannot be recognized due to strong hyperchromasia. Since the specimen was collected mechanically, many destroyed cells can be seen. (X400, Pap.)
(c) Histologic specimen. Lymph-like hyperchromatic cells proliferate infiltratively in submucosa. (X200, H.E.)
(d) Chest X-ray film. The primary lesion is located in the left middle lung field. Findings of mediastinal lymph node involvement are prominent. Rapid lymph node involvement is clinically characteristic of small cell carcinoma.

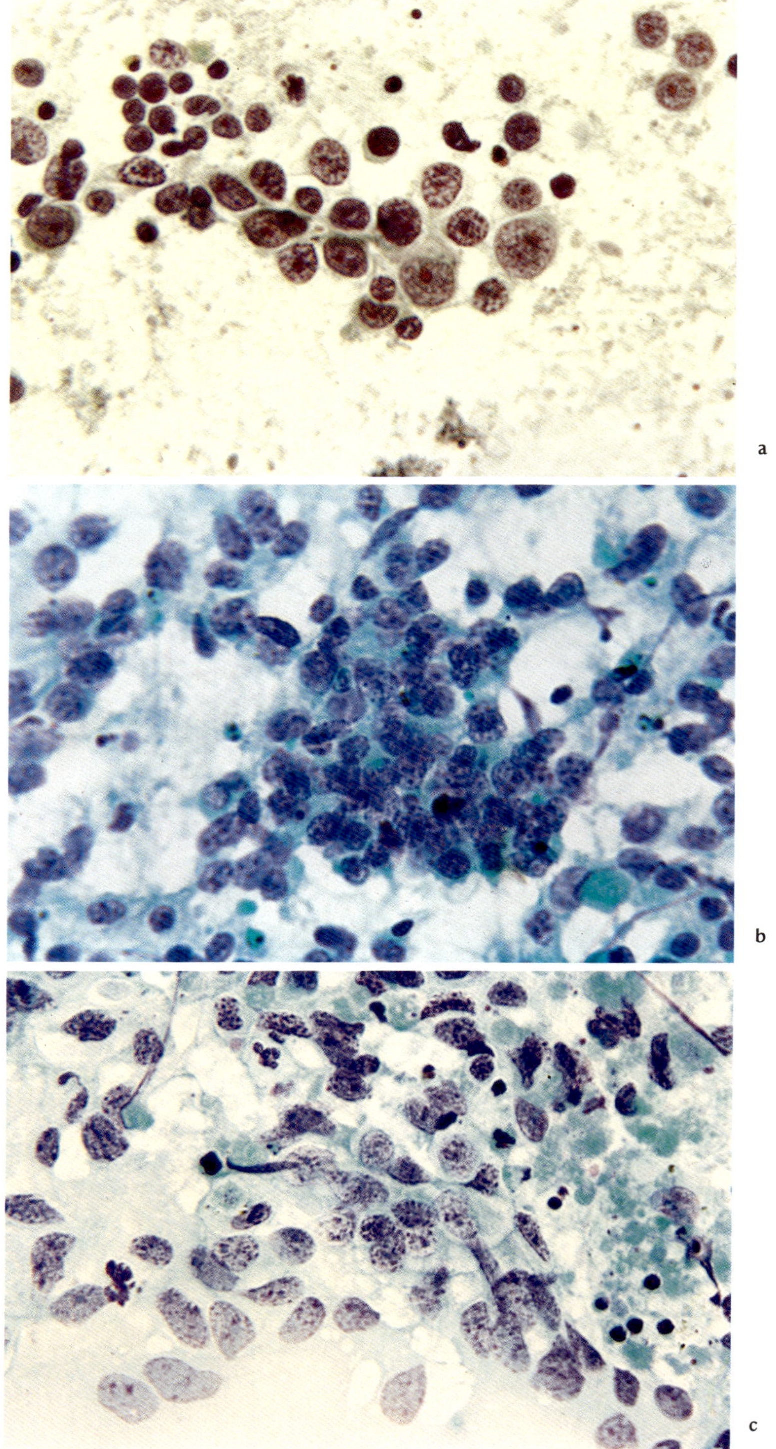

Fig. 112　See legend on opposite page.

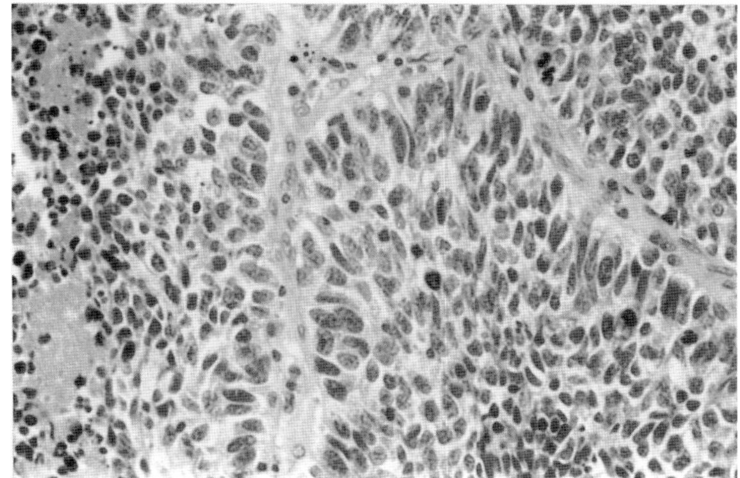

Fig. 112 Small cell carcinoma, intermediate cell type.
(a)   Sputum cytology specimen. The cells are polygonal and have more abundant cytoplasm than oat cell type cells. Several nucleoli can be observed. (X400, Pap.)
(b)   Brushing cytology specimen. The cluster of cells shows superimposition and adhesion with destroyed materials resulting from the mechanical method of harvesting the specimen. Compared to oat cell type cells, the cells are large and show a greater variation in size. These carcinoma cells possess frothy basophilically staining cytoplasm, the border of which is usually unclear. The intranuclear structure is finely granular. Small nucleoli are recognizable. (X400, Pap.)
(c)   Needle aspiration cytology specimen. Polygonal, larger polyhedral cells are seen. Hyperchromasia is less prominent than oat cell type. Intranuclear structure is clearer than in oat cell type. Chromatin is granular, multinucleoli are seen and the cytoplasm is abundant and frothy. (X400, Pap.)
(d)   Histologic specimen. This type of small cell carcinoma is composed of polygonal cells with somewhat larger polyhedral hyperchromatic nuclei. (X400, H.E.)

ADENOCARCINOMA

Since many tumors of this histologic type originate in subsegmental or more distal bronchi, it can sometimes be detected at an early stage on the basis of an abnormal shadow on chest X-ray film (Fig. 113c). However, by the same token, in cases of peripheral origin, cells are rarely recognized in sputum specimens; therefore, the most suitable diagnostic approach is to perform brushing or percutaneous needle cytology under X-ray television guidance. Nevertheless, a small number of adenocarcinomas can arise in large bronchi, originating from the mucous gland. This type of adenocarcinoma shows glandular formation and often produces mucin. The authors divide adenocarcinoma into well differentiated (Fig. 113b), poorly differentiated (Fig. 114) and bronchioloalveolar types (Figs. 115c, 116b and 117b) on the basis of cell features.

Clinical Findings: (Chest X-ray) Adenocarcinoma develops mainly in the periphery of the lung. In such cases, it is generally easy to detect the round tumor shadow in the chest X-ray film. The shadow is usually accompanied by notching, spicules and indentation of the pleura.
(Fiberoptic Bronchoscopy) In the case of peripheral tumors usually no abnormal findings are observed endoscopically. However, frequently adenocarcinoma originating in larger bronchi reveals submucosal tumor proliferation with engorgement of neoplastic vessels.

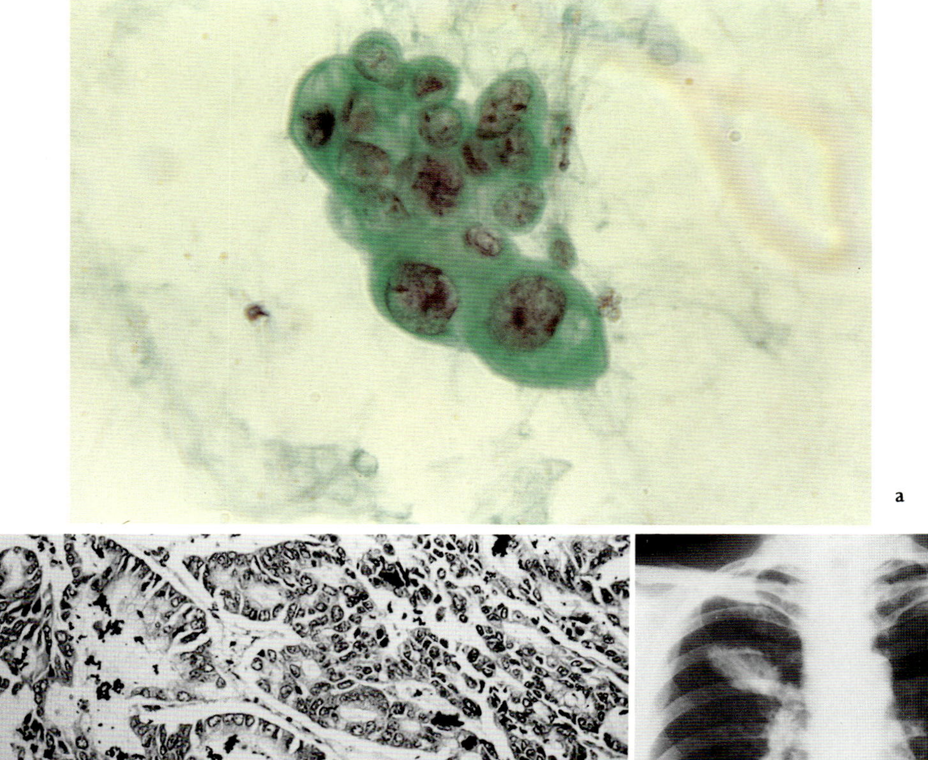

Fig. 113 Well differentiated adenocarcinoma.
(a)   Sputum cytology specimen. The cells show a papillary arrangement with a strong tendency to overlap. Vacuoles can be seen in the basophilically staining cytoplasm of the cells. Large round nucleoli are present and the nucleus is off-centered. (X400, Pap.)
(b)   Histologic findings. Polymorphic cancer cells forming tubules can be seen. (X200, H.E.)
(c)   Chest X-ray findings of a 38-year-old woman showing a well defined oval tumor shadow in the right upper lung field.

Well Differentiated

Sputum cytology specimens

In sputum specimens, well differentiated adenocarcinoma cells tend to appear in clusters more often than do squamous cell carcinoma cells. There is remarkable overlapping within the clusters and occasional papillary and tubular formation (Figs. 113a and 118a).

The cells are rounded or oval, and the variation in size is remarkable. The cytoplasm stains *light green* with small vacuoles, and large mucin vacuoles are

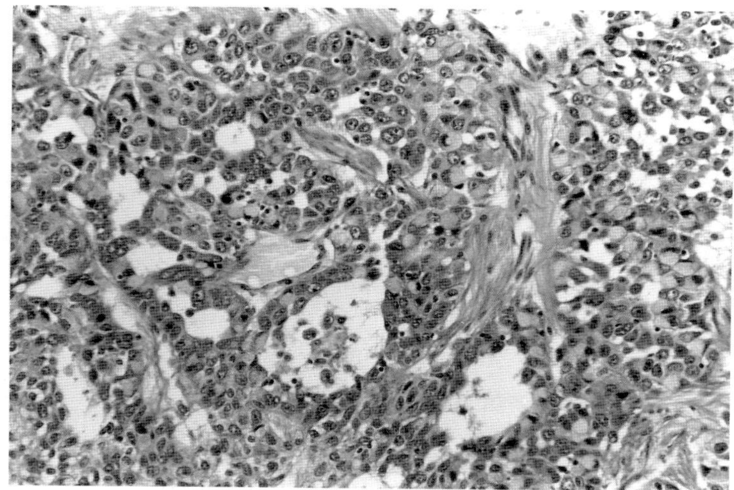

Fig. 114 Poorly differentiated adenocarcinoma. Tubular formation was seen in only a few parts of the entire specimen. This histologic specimen is composed mostly of cells with mucin in their cytoplasm. (X200, H.E.)

occasionally seen. PAS stain proves the mucus content. The nucleus is displaced to the edge of the cell border by the vacuoles.

The nucleus is circular or rounded with a thin nuclear membrane, and in degenerated specimens the nuclear borders show irregular folds. The nucleus is displaced to the edge of the cell, and clusters of cells with nuclei displaced to peripheral portions of the cytoplasm are a typical finding.

The chromatin is granular, and the more degenerated the cells are, the greater the tendency is for the granularity of the chromatin to progress from fine to coarse (Hattori, 1979). The chromatin does not tend to collect at the nuclear margins. When cells appear in clusters, differences in the chromatin pattern and hyperchromasia of the individual cells can be recognized.

Nucleoli, typically large and round, are often observed at the centers of the nuclei.

Brushing and needle cytology specimens

Specimens obtained by brushing and needle cytology technique in cases of well differentiated adenocarcinoma usually show clusters with a strong tendency to overlap. However, typical papillary formation frequently observed in sputum specimens has a tendency to be destroyed in brushing and needle cytology specimens.

The typically clear cytoplasm shows a basophilic staining pattern, with tiny vacuoles giving it the appearance of lace, and large vacuoles are not commonly seen. The round nuclei have smooth nuclear membranes. Although the nuclear chromatin is usually finely granular, it becomes coarser as the degeneration becomes more advanced. The nucleoli are large, rounded and occasionally acidophilic and usually are located centrally in the nucleus (Figs. 118b, 119 and 120).

Well differentiated adenocarcinoma cells must also be differentiated from atypical hyperplastic columnar cells and atypical hyperplastic basal cells. The

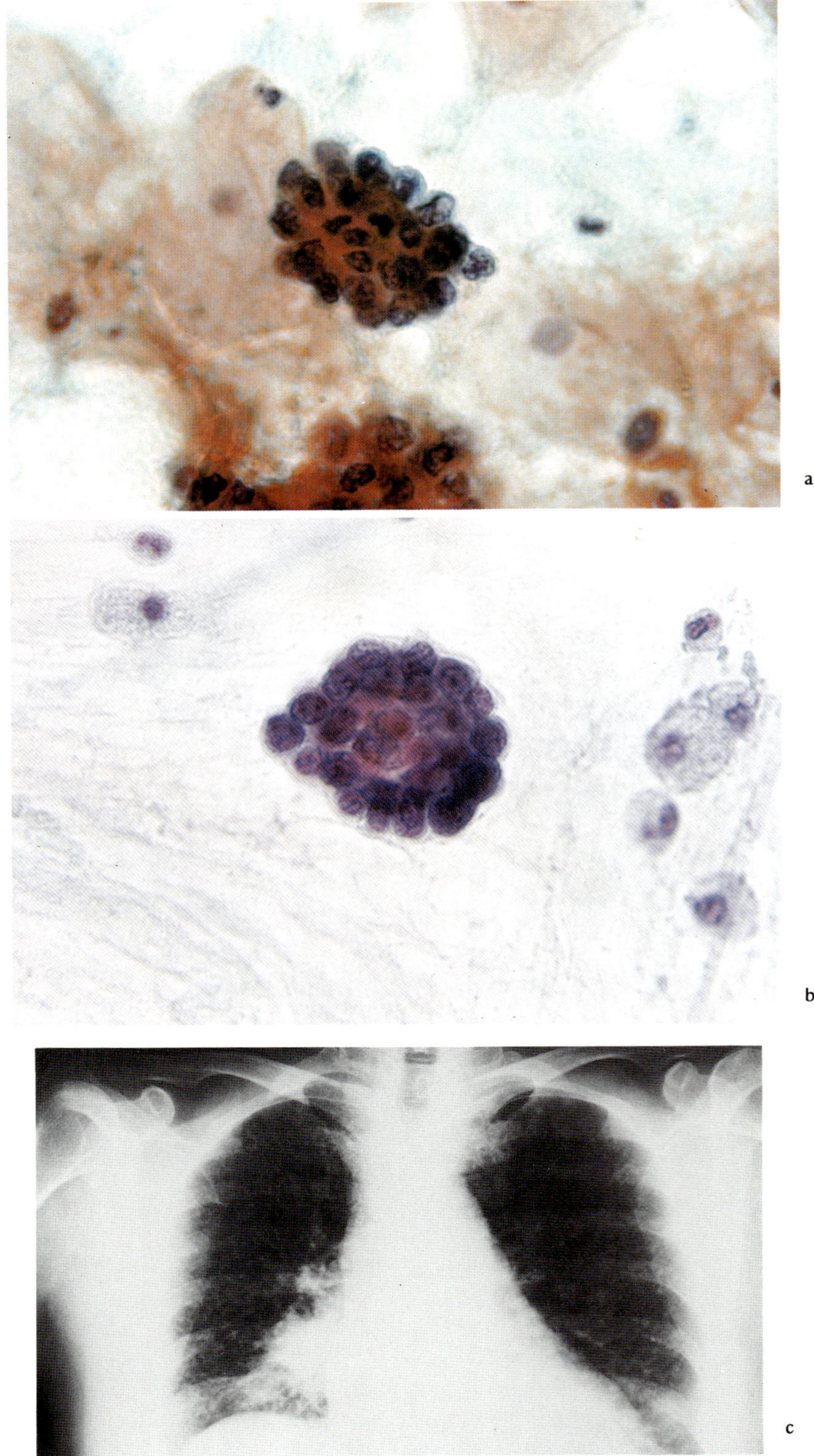

Fig. 115   See legend on opposite page.

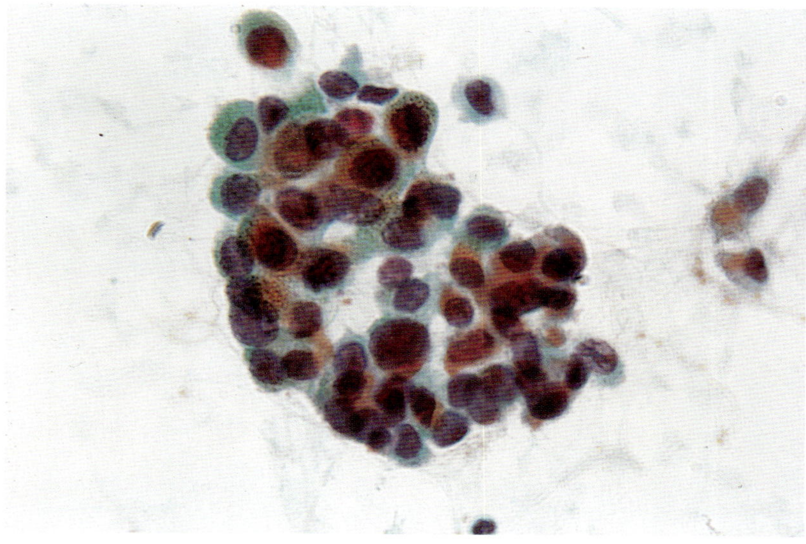

a

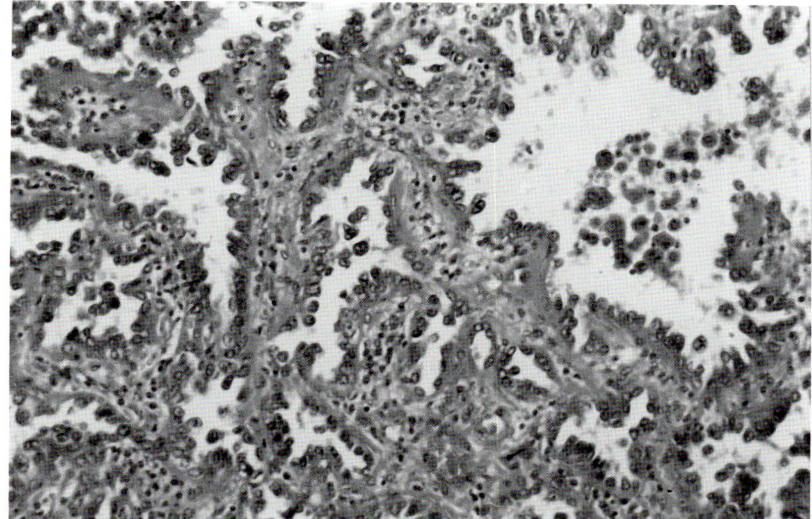

b

Fig. 116 Bronchioloalveolar cell carcinoma.
(a)   Needle aspiration cytology specimen. The small cuboidal cells in relatively loose clusters show hyperchromasia with well stained basophilic cytoplasm. Variation in nuclear size and shape are observed. Diagnostic features are the cuboidal cell and the prominent nucleoli. (X400, Pap.)
(b)   Histologic findings. Cuboidal cancer cells proliferate alongside bronchioloalveolar walls. (X200, H.E.)

Fig. 115 Bronchioloalveolar cell carcinoma.
(a)   Sputum cytology specimen. The tightly packed cluster of cells shows a high degree of differentiation while the variation in nuclear size is low. Irregular nuclear shape can be seen. Chromatin is not particularly dense. (X400, Pap.)
(b)   Brushing cytology specimen. The small cells are packed in a compact cluster. The cytoplasm is scanty and the nuclear size is variable. Chromatin is coarse and nucleoli are observed. (X400, Pap.)
(c)   Chest X-ray findings of a 60-year-old woman. Multiple diffuse lesions are recognized in both lungs.

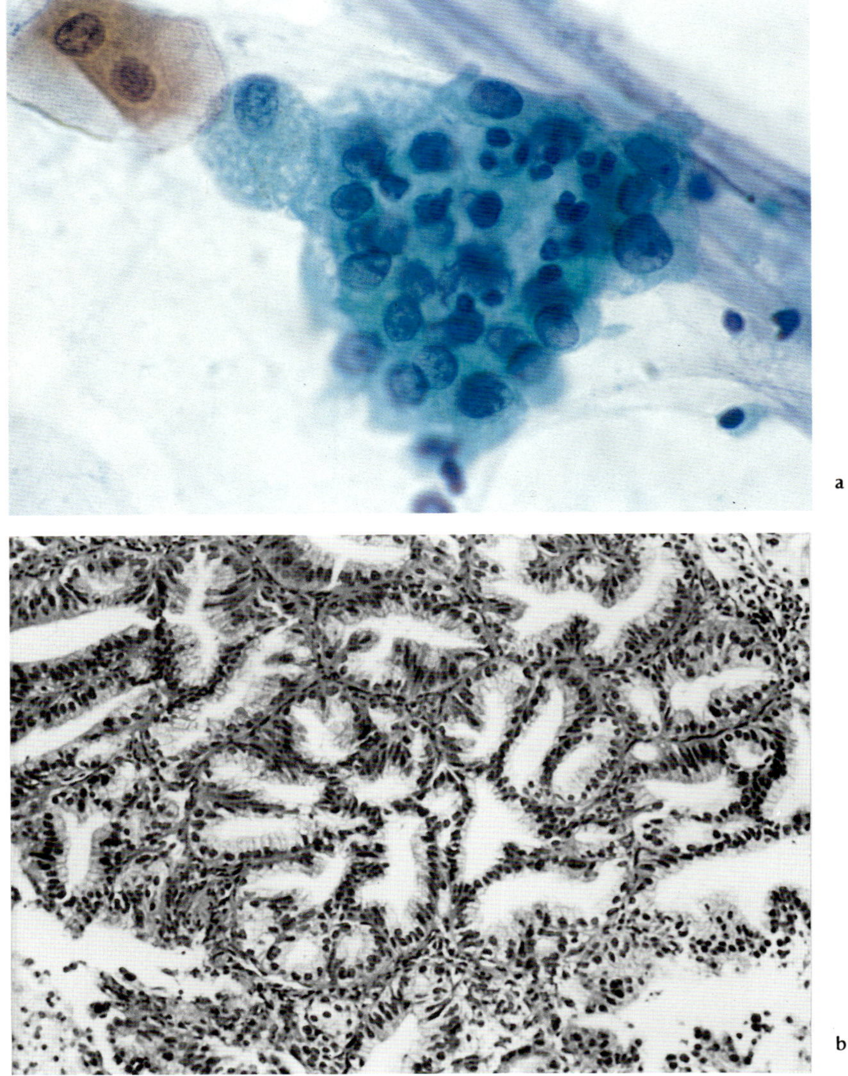

Fig. 117 Bronchioloalveolar cell carcinoma.
(a) Sputum cytology specimen. The cells in the cluster are composed of round or oval nuclei with abundant cytoplasm. The cytoplasm contains mucus. (X400, Pap.)
(b) Histologic findings. A single layer of tall columnar cancer cells is seen proliferating along the alveolar wall. (x200, H.E.)

latter cells display ciliation and terminal plate or homogeneous intranuclear chromatin patterns. Adenocarcinoma cells frequently show smooth nuclear membrane and prominent round and large nucleoli that allow their differentiation from benign lesions.

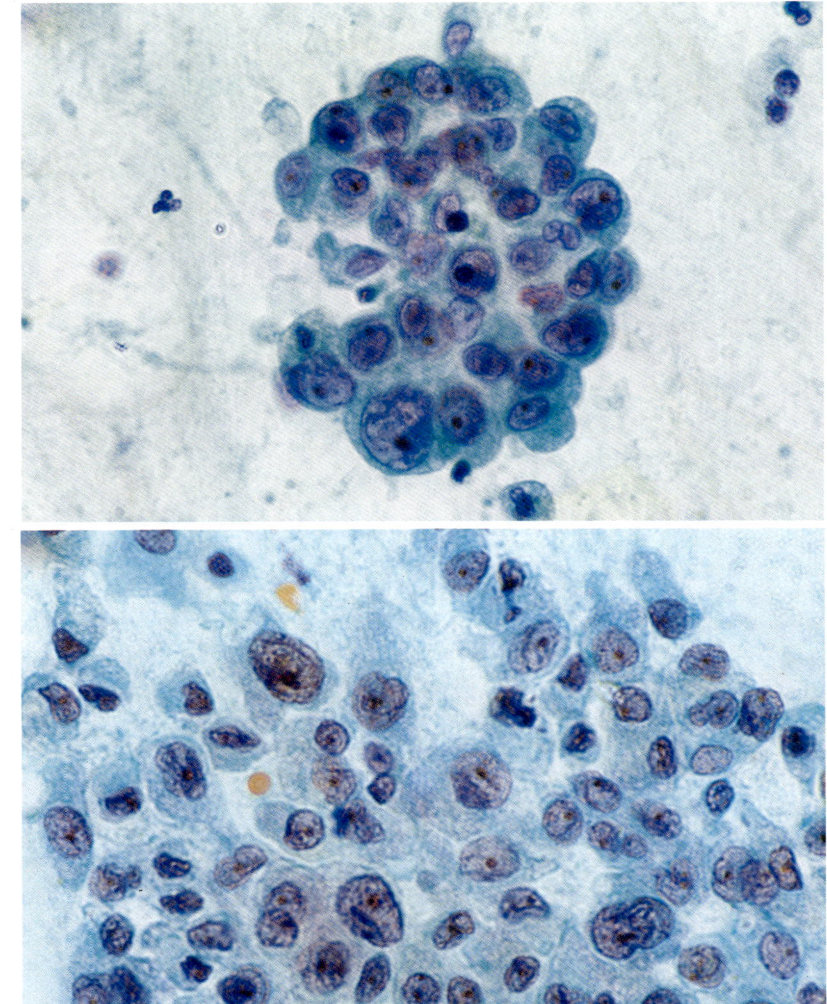

Fig. 118 Well differentiated adenocarcinoma.
(a) Sputum cytology specimen. A large papillary cluster with overlapping round cells is seen. Hyperchromasia is not striking. Nucleoli are round and prominent. (X400, Pap.)
(b) Brushing cytology specimen. The typical papillary arrangement is destroyed in the brushing cytology specimen. However the clear cytoplasm with tiny vacuoles, prominent round nucleoli and finely granular chromatin pattern can be recognized as characteristic of adenocarcinoma cells. (X400, Pap.)

Poorly Differentiated

Sputum cytology specimens

Poorly differentiated adenocarcinoma in sputum specinens usually appears as single cells, unlike the cells of well differentiated adenocarcinoma, but when the cells do appear in clusters, they display a slight tendency to overlap. The

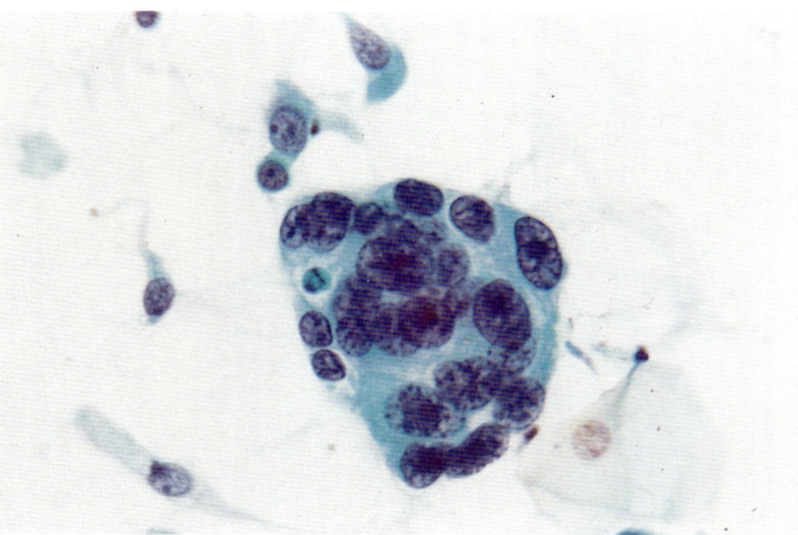

Fig. 119 Well differentiated adenocarcinoma in a brushing cytology specimen. A cluster with a tendency to overlap can be seen. The round nuclei have smooth nuclear membranes and large and rounded nucleoli are located at the peripheral portions of the cytoplasm. Some nuclei show hyperchromasia and coarse chromatin. (X400, Pap.)

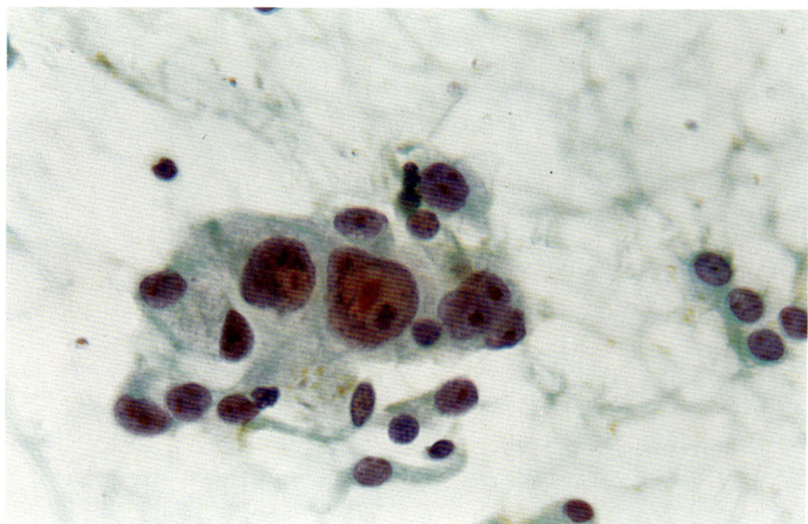

Fig. 120 Well differentiated adenocarcinoma in a needle aspiration cytology specimen. Variation in nuclear size, hyperchromasia, prominent nucleoli and frothy cytoplasm suggest adenocarcinoma. (X400, Pap.)

cytoplasm is fragile and shows the tendency of cyanophilic staining, but some cells demonstrate eosinophilic staining as a result of degeneration, which also induces the formation of small vacuoles. The nuclei are more polygonal than those in well differentiated specimens. The nuclear margins are smooth, and the nuclei of most cells show coarsely granular chromatin. Typically, one or more round nucleoli are present, and there is usually little displacement of the nucleus. The diagnosis of adenocarcinoma can be made on the basis of the presence of vacuolated cytoplasm, overlapping of cells and the presence of one or more round nucleoli (Fig. 121a, b).

Brushing and needle cytology specimens

The degree of degeneration of fresh specimens of poorly differentiated adenocarcinoma is understandably lower than that in sputum specimens, and the cytoplasm shows basophilic staining. The cells often appear in large clusters and show overlapping. Apart from the overlapping, the clusters show few of the characteristics of adenocarcinoma, as seen in sputum specimens. The cytoplasm is frothy, and demarcation of cellular borders is difficult. The nuclei are either rounded or polygonal with smooth and thin margins. The chromatin is either finely or coarsely granular, and a few nucleoli are frequently observed.

The cellular overlapping, the lacy cytoplasmic pattern and the round nucleoli are the only distinguishing characteristics of poorly differentiated adenocarcinoma (Fig. 121c—e).

In many cases, it is difficult to distinguish between poorly differentiated adenocarcinoma, poorly differentiated squamous cell carcinoma and large cell carcinoma. The mild degree of cellular overlapping, hyperchromasia, irregular aggregation of chromatin along the nuclear margins, irregularly shaped nucleoli, are diagnostic features of poorly differentiated squamous cell carcinoma, whereas the presence of large cells, several nucleoli, loss of cellular adherence, and weak stainability of the nuclei permit the diagnosis of large cell carcinoma.

Bronchioloalveolar Type

Bronchioloalveolar cell carcinoma is a special form of adenocarcinoma in which the tumor cells proliferate along the walls of the pulmonary alveoli without displaying remarkable destruction. It is thought to originate in terminal bronchi or alveoli regardless of the nature of tumor cells.

Sputum cytology specimens

Differentiation of bronchioloalveolar cell carcinoma from bronchogenic adenocarcinoma is possible using sputum materials (Roger et al., 1976). Cells shows a strong tendency to overlap and frequently appear in papillary clumps. Usually the cells are small and oval. Cytoplasm is scanty and usually clear but sometimes partially acidophilic. Occasionally several small vacuoles can be recognized, but large vacuoles are infrequent except in extremely degenerated cells. Nucleoli are generally, small, rounded and exhibit homogeneous chromatin. In cells with several vacuoles the nucleoli exhibit a tendency to be displaced towards the periphery of the nuclei (Figs. 115a and 117a).

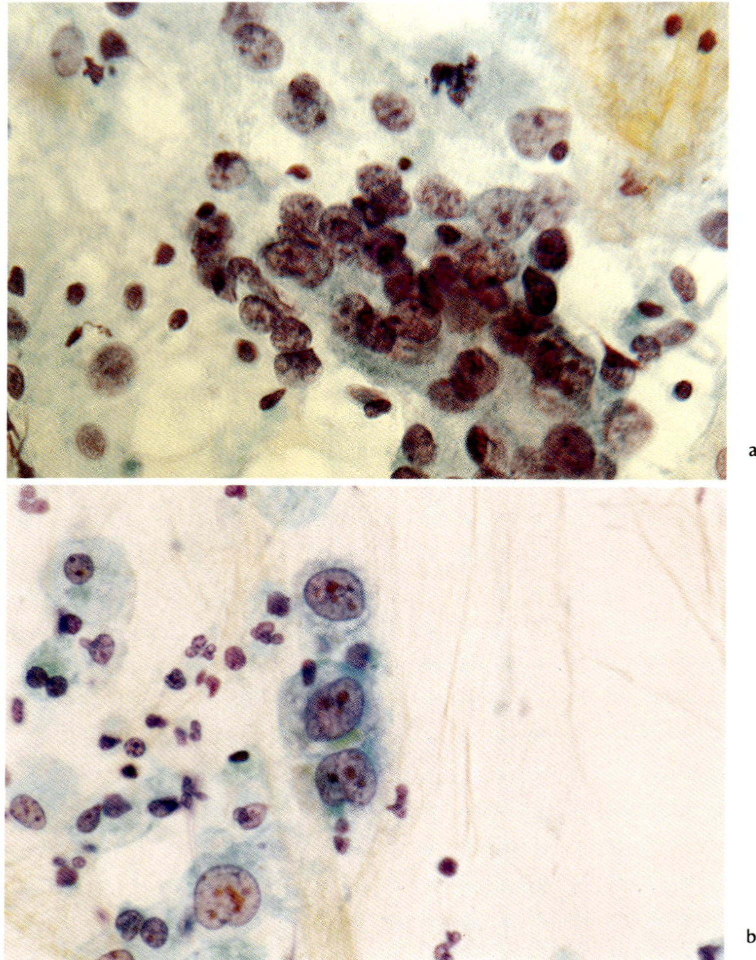

Fig. 121 Poorly differentiated adenocarcinoma.
(a) Sputum cytology specimen. Cells with increased N/C ratio can be seen in loose clusters. The round nucleus has distinct nucleoli. The coarsely granular chromatin and the basophilic cytoplasm are suspicious of adenocarcinoma. (X400, Pap.)
(b) Sputum cytology specimen. The cells with poor cellular adherence, fragile basophilic cytoplasm, irregular nuclear shape, multiple nucleoli are seen. Chromatin is finely granular. The diagnostic features in adenocarcinoma are nucleoli and vacuolated cytoplasm. (X400, Pap.)
(c) Brushing cytology specimen. The cluster of cells shows overlapping and glandular formation is not recognizable. Hyperchromatic nuclei with variable nuclear size are seen. The round or oval nuclei possess large nucleoli and no clumps of chromatin can be seen along the nuclear border. Prominent nucleoli are suspicious of adenocarcinoma. (X400, Pap.)
(d) Brushing cytology specimen. The nuclear chromatin is finely granular and several nucleoli can be recognized. The nuclear border is smooth and some nuclei show hyperchromasia. Cytoplasm stains frothily. Although it is difficult to make a diagnosis of adenocarcinoma from these findings, the frothy cytoplasm and light nuclei are suggestive diagnostic features. (x400, Pap.)
(e) Needle cytology specimen showing a cell cluster with abundant frothy cytoplasm. Hyperchromasia is not striking. Irregular nucleoli are seen in some nuclei. The frothy, vacuolated cytoplasm and light nuclei are diagnostic features. (x400, Pap.)

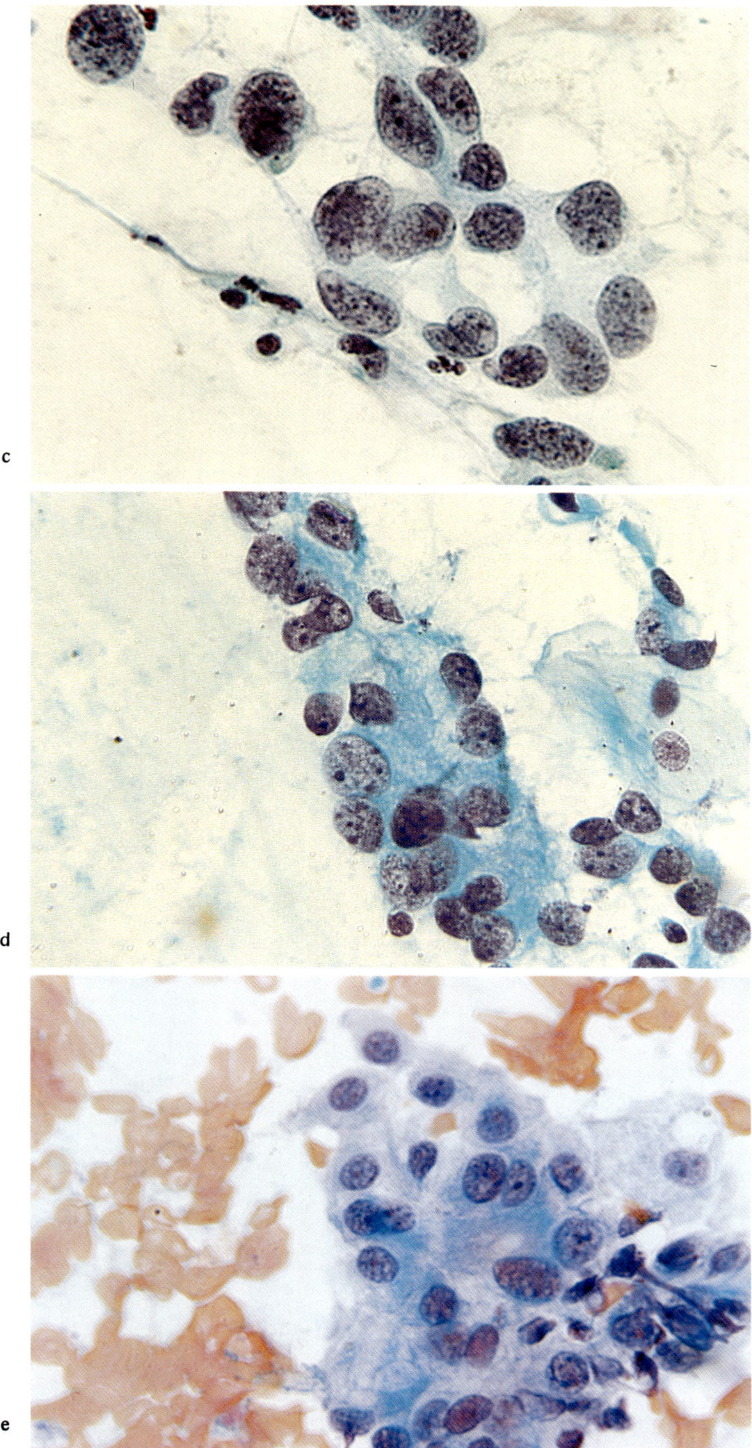

Fig. 121 See legend on opposite page.

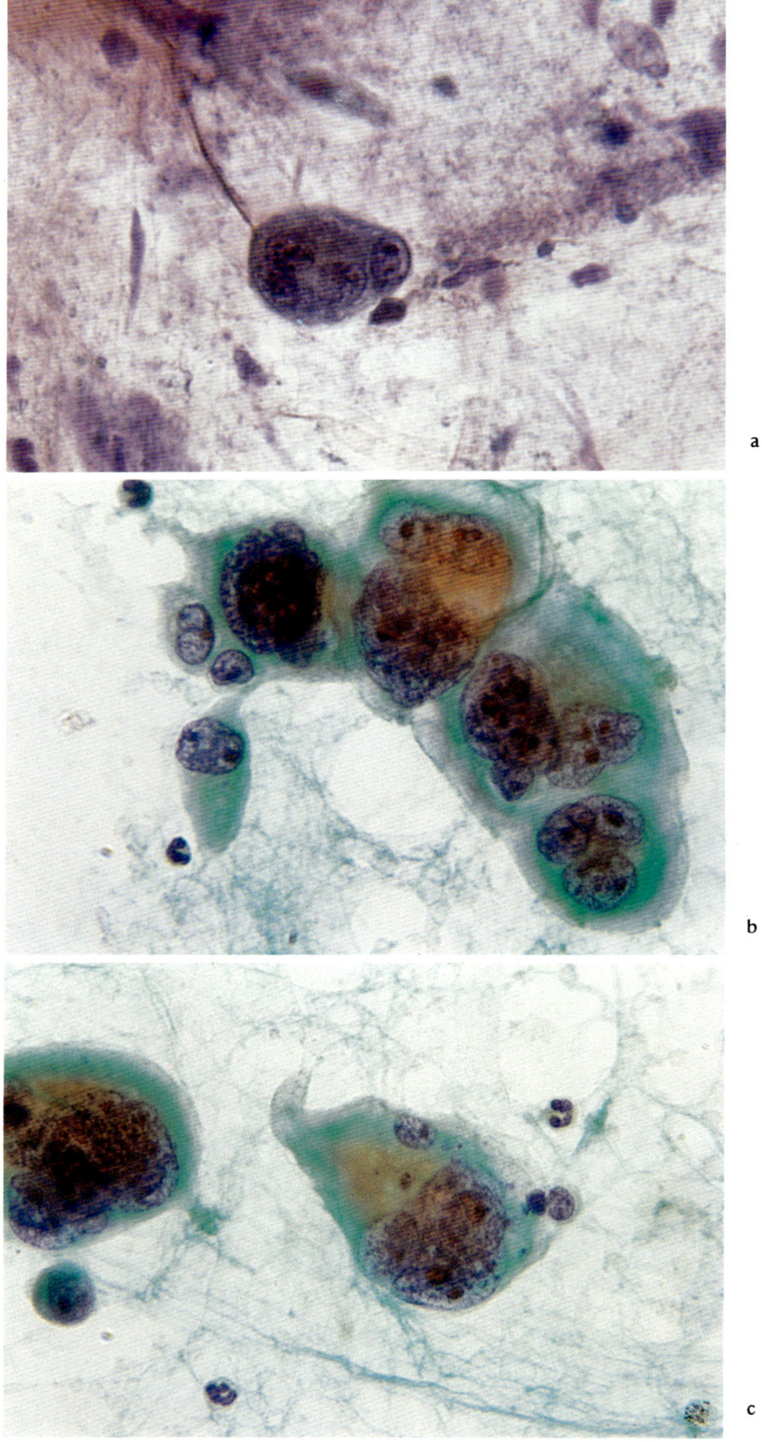

Fig. 122   See legend on opposite page.

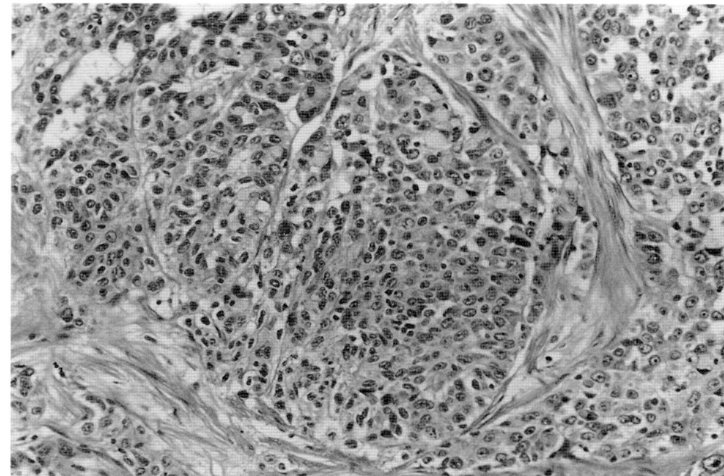

Fig. 122 Large cell carcinoma.
(a) Sputum cytology specimen. The large cells with pale blue basophilic cytoplasm appear in loose
     clusters or as single cells. Large vacuoles are seen in the cytoplasm. Nucleoli are large and
     irregular. (X400, Pap.)
(b) Brushing cytology specimen. The cells, appearing as a loose cluster, are large with frothy baso-
     philic cytoplasm. The nucleoli have relative smooth borders and finely to coarsely granular
     chromatin. Large nucleoli are prominent. (X400, Pap.)
(c) Transbronchial aspiration cytology specimen. Large cells with large rounded nuclei and frothy
     basophilic cytoplasm can be seen. Nucleoli are large, irregular in shape and sometimes are
     multiple. Cellular adhesion is low.
(d) Histologic findings. This type of tumor does not show any tendency to differentiate. Cancer
     cells proliferate in a solid nest. (X200, H.E.)

Brushing and needle cytology specimens

Most of the specimens obtained by these methods show the same degree of tightly
packed clusters, but cells appear frequently in sheets or as single cells. Cytoplasm
is relatively abundant, some cells with vacuolation show weak basophilia. Nuclei
are small, rounded and have a smooth border. Chromatin is granular and many
cells show a homogeneous distribution. Variation in cellular size and shape is less
than that of bronchogenic adenocarcinoma (Figs. 115b and 116a).

In terms of differential diagnosis it is important to differentiate such cells from
hyperplastic columnar epithelium. The differential point is the presence of cilia at
the margin of clusters in hyperplastic columnar cells (see Fig. 64).

LARGE CELL CARCINOMA

The cells of large cell carcinoma do not show any differentiated characteristics
such as squamous cell carcinoma or adenocarcinoma. This tumor appears as a
collection of large, undifferentiated carcinoma cells. It tends to originate distal to
segmental bronchi, frequently appearing on X-ray films as a tumor shadow in the
lung field (Fig. 122e). Clinically large cell carcinoma displays a strong tendency to
metastasize and has a poor prognosis.

The cytoplasm stains in a variety of ways, and the nucleoli are usually prominent (Fig. 123d). A much larger so-called giant cell can sometimes be seen. The giant cell subtype of large cell carcinoma is defined as a tumor in which 30% or more of the cells are mononuclear or multinuclear giant cells (Fig. 122d).

Clinical Findings: (Chest X-ray) Roentgenologically this histologic type closely resembles squamous cell carcinoma. However, it shows a tendency to originate in a slightly more peripheral location, therefore its appearance as a mass in the lung field is slightly more frequent.
(Fiberoptic Bronchoscopy) The tumor appears frequently as a polypoid tumor.

Sputum cytology specimens

In sputum specimens, the cells appear either singly or as loose clusters with little overlapping. The cells are large and usually round or oval. The cytoplasm typically shows pale blue cyanophilic staining, although eosinophilic staining cells are sometimes seen. The borders of the fragile cytoplasm are unclear, and large vacuoles are sometimes observed. The nuclei are typically located in the center of the cells and are usually round or oval. The chromatin is coarsely granular, and thickened irregular nuclear membranes are seen. Some of the one or more irregularly shaped nucleoli usually recognized are occasionally dramatically increased in size (Fig. 123a).

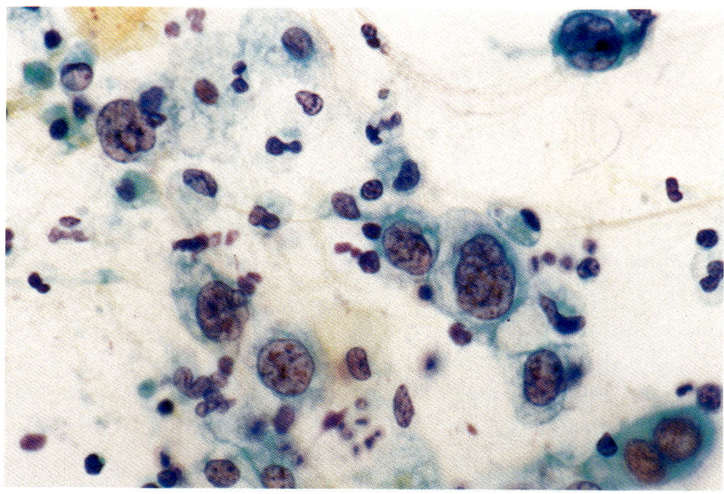

Fig. 123   Large cell carcinoma, giant cell type.
(a)   Sputum cytology specimen. A multinucleated giant cell with coarsely granular chromatin can be seen. Generally single cells appear in sputum in this type of tumor. (X400, Pap.)
(b)   Brushing cytology specimen. Multinucleated giant cells with large vacuoles in cytoplasm can be observed. Single or multiple nucleoli are observed, and chromatin in small cells is coarsely granular. (X400, Pap.)
(c)   Needle cytology specimen showing single multinucleated giant cells with abundant well staining cytoplasm. (X400, Pap.)
(d)   Histologic findings. Bizarre, large cells, some with multinuclei proliferate solidly. Adhesion of cells is low. (X200, H.E.)
(e)   Chest X-ray findings of a 52-year-old man. Well defined tumor shadow in the left hilum is seen. This type of tumor has a tendency to develop in relatively large bronchi.

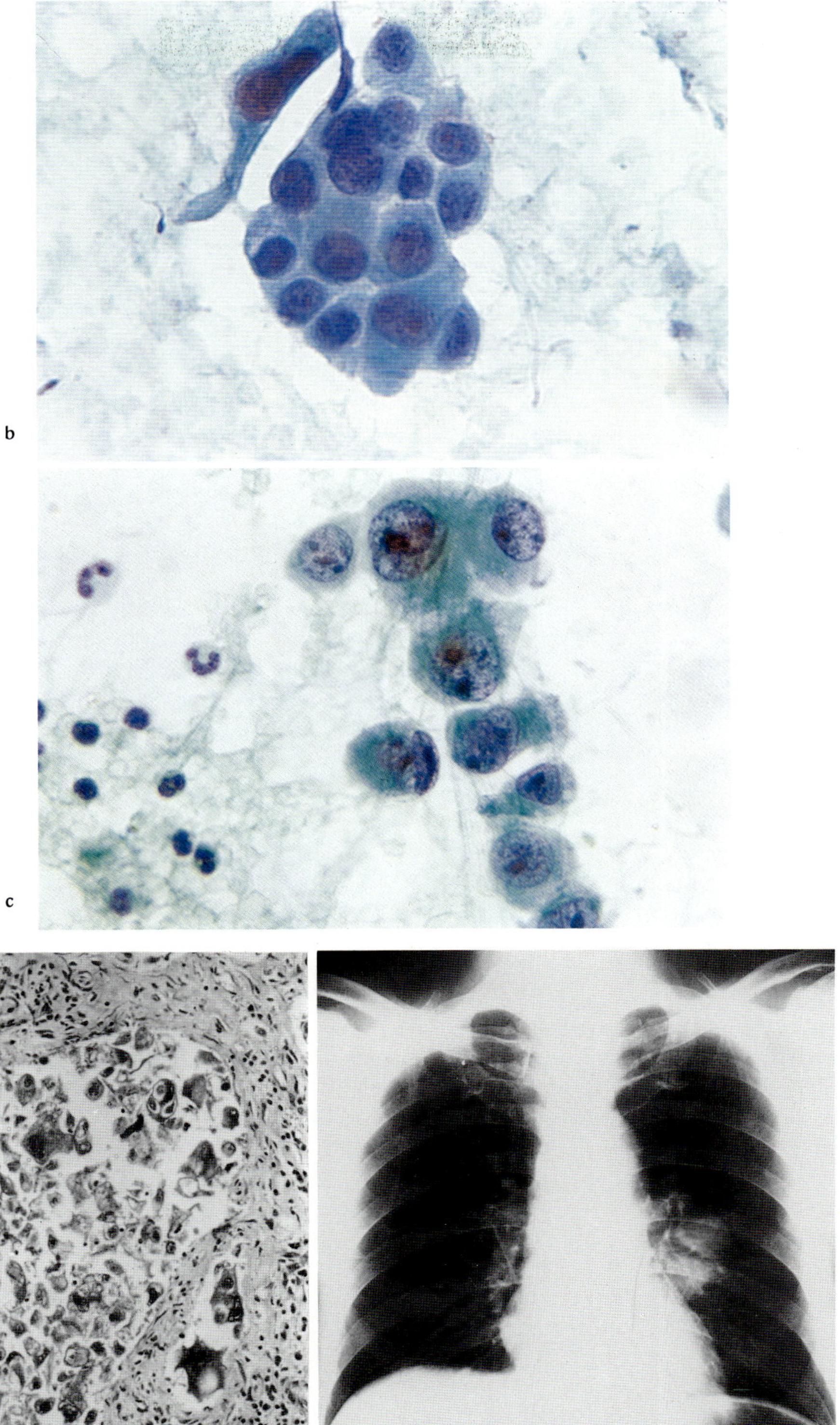

Fig. 123   See legend on opposite page.

Giant cell carcinoma appears as individual cells in sputum specimens. The mononuclear or multinuclear cells are large and round or irregularly shaped. The cytoplasm stains in a variety of ways and sometimes contains large vacuoles. The nuclei are round or oval, with coarsely granular chromatin. The irregularly shaped nucleoli are generally situated at the center of the nucleus. Cytophagocytosis is occasionally observed (Fig. 122a).

Brushing and needle cytology specimens
The most frequent appearance is as loose clusters. The fragile cytoplasm of the large cells is frothy and exhibits basophilic staining. Vacuoles are sometimes seen in the cytoplasm, with indistinct borders. The nuclei have relatively smooth borders and unevenly distributed, finely to coarsely granular chromatin. Most nucleoli are large, round or irregular in shape (Fig. 123b, c).

Giant cell carcinoma is more often observed in fresh specimens than in sputum specimens, in which it is easily diagnosed because of its characteristic appearance (Sawada et al., 1981) as described above in the *Sputum Cytology* section (Fig. 122b, c).

Since large cell carcinoma cells show resemblance to the cells of poorly differentiated squamous cell carcinoma or to poorly differentiated adenocarcinoma, differential diagnosis is frequently difficult. Large cell carcinoma may be differentiated from poorly differentiated adenocarcinoma on the basis of the low degree of cellular overlapping, the irregularity of the nucleoli and the presence of coarsely granular chromatin, but the characteristic features for distinguishing large cell carcinoma from poorly differentiated squamous cell carcinoma are the presence of multilobed giant cells and stainability of the cytoplasm in the case of the former.

ADENOSQUAMOUS CARCINOMA

Adenosquamous carcinoma is a relatively infrequent type possessing both squamous and acinar or papillary differentiaction. A diagnosis of combined form should be made only when the minority type occupies 20% or more of the entire cut surface of the histological specimen. When both adenocarcinoma cells and squamous cell carcinoma cells are observed in sputum the possibility of two tumors, one of each histological type must be considered. It can also be difficult to make a differential diagnosis between these histologic types by sputum cytology only. Brushing cytology obtained from a certain focus facilitates the establishment of a cytologic diagnosis of adenosquamous if both cells are observed at the same time.

CARCINOID

Carcinoid is believed to derive from Kulchitsky cells of the bronchial gland (Bensch et al., 1965). Cells of this type rarely appear in sputum cytology but can be recognized if the lesion originates centrally with mucosal invasion (Fig. 124c—e) (Kato, 1982).

Clinical Findings: (Chest X-ray) This tumor generally originates in the large bronchi. Therefore, the tumor shadow appears in the hilar region. Tumor shadow is sometimes accompanied by a secondary infiltrative shadow and/or atelectasis.
(Fiberoptic Bronchoscopy) The tumor usually develops submucosally, therefore the tumor surface is smooth with polypoid proliferation.

Sputum cytology specimens

Since it frequently proliferates covered by normal bronchial mucosa, carcinoid cells rarely appear in sputum at an early stage. However, as the lesion increases in size, it can break through the normal mucosa, in which case it can be seen in sputum cytology specimens. Carcinoid cells in sputum specimens are larger than lymphocytes and have more abundant and frothy cytoplasm with rounded nuclei and one or two clearly discernible nucleoli and granular chromatin. In sputum specimens, carcinoid cells often appear as single cells. Carcinoid cells can be distinguished from histiocytes due to the lack of phagocytic function and clearly discernible nucleoli of the former, from lymphocytes on the basis of the quantity of cytoplasm and from small cell carcinoma cells on the basis of the amount of chromatin (Fig. 124a).

Brushing and needle cytology specimens

Cells obtained directly from carcinoid lesions are larger than those observed in sputum specimens. The abundant cytoplasm stains light blue-green. The nuclear chromatin is finely granular, and nucleoli can be clearly recognized. Cellular adhesion is weak (Figs. 124b and 125). Cellular arrangement shows sheet-like patterns. These cells must be distinguished from intermediate type small cell carcinoma, and basal cell hyperplasia.

MUCOEPIDERMOID CARCINOMA

This tumor derives from the bronchial gland and frequently occurs near lobular bronchi, developing endobronchially as a polypoid lesion. It is a rare tumor that possesses both solid epidermoid foci and glandular histologic features (Fig. 126e-g). This tumor, which shows invasive growth and distant metastasis (Sniffen et al., 1958; Meckstroth et al., 1961) is occasionally covered by the bronchial mucosa, and thus in such cases cells rarely appears in sputum, TBAC is the most effective method in establishing a definitive diagnosis.

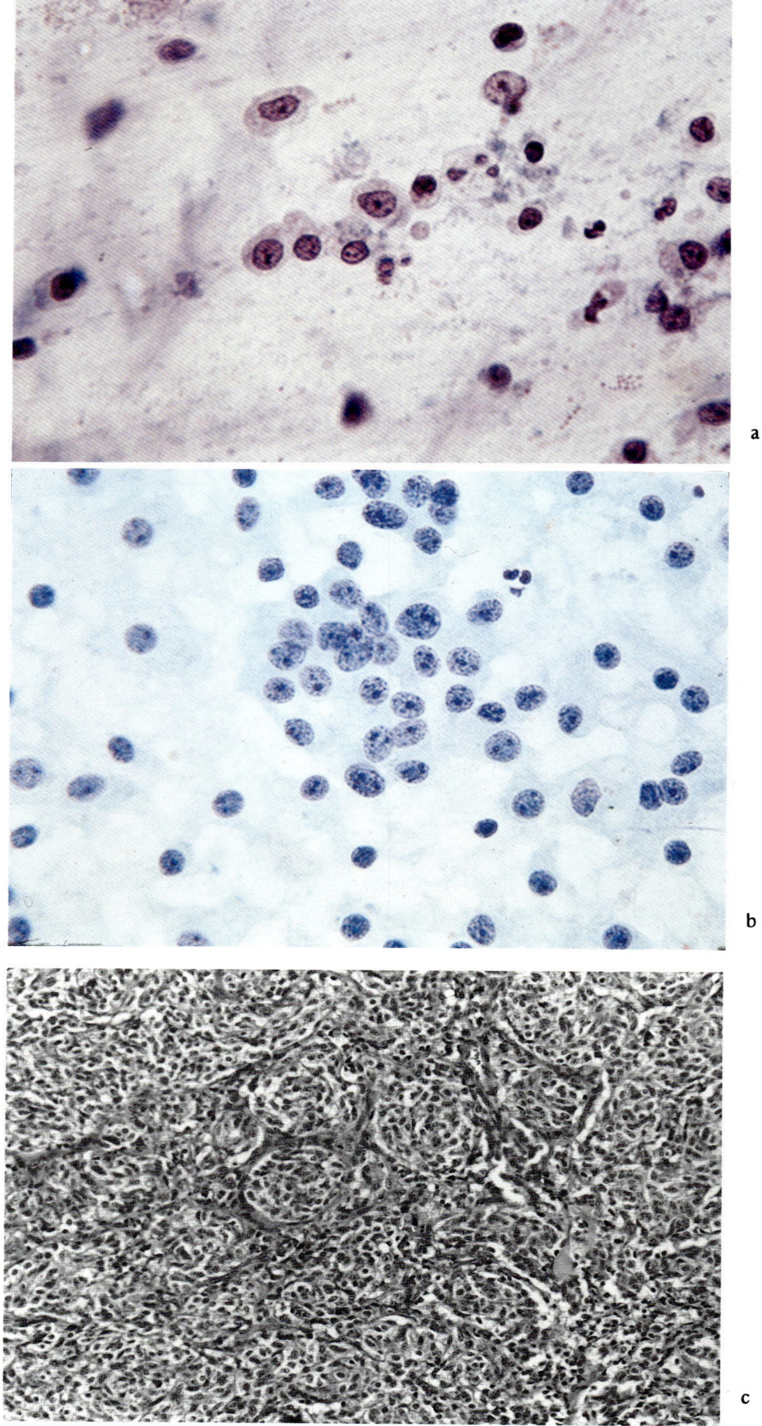

Fig. 124   See legend on opposite page.

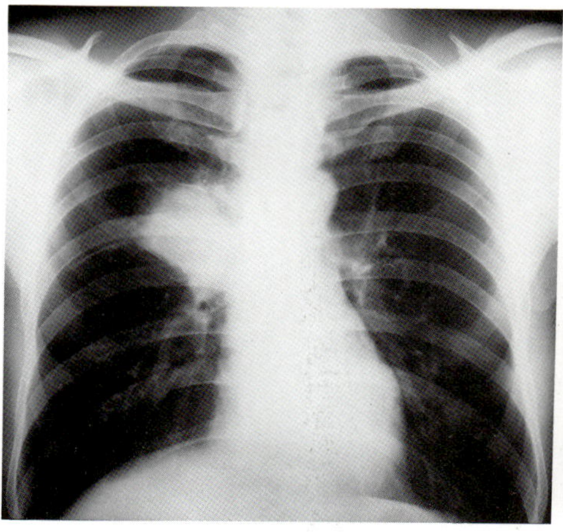
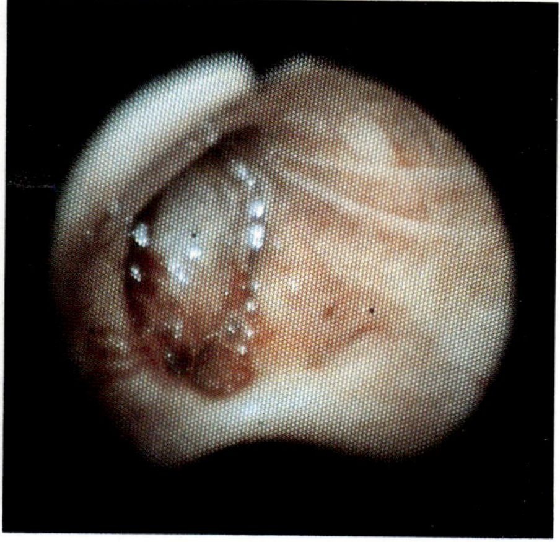

Fig. 124 Carcinoid.
(a) Sputum cytology specimen. Carcinoid cells are larger than lymphocytes and are about the same size as columnar cells. The cytoplasm is relatively abundant and frothy. The nucleus is rounded and has roughly granular chromatin. The round nucleoli are clearly recognizable. Caution must be exercised to distinguish carcinoid cells from histiocytes, lymphocytes and small cell carcinoma. (X400, Pap.)
(b) Brushing cytology specimen. Intracellular adhesion is weak and the abundant cytoplasm weakly stains light green. The border of the cytoplasm of many cells is unclear and the round-to-oval nuclei possess thin and irregular membranes. The size of the nucleus is generally approximately that of columnar cells, but occasionally a wide variation in nuclear size can be observed. Chromatin is granular and the amount of chromatin does not appear to be significantly increased. One or more nucleoli are usually present. (X400, Pap.)
(c) Histologic findings. This tumor is composed of cells with small, round nuclei and abundant eosinophilic cytoplasm. (X200, H.E.)
(d) Chest X-ray findings of a 55-year-old man. A well defined round tumor shadow can be seen in the right hilum.
(e) Fiberoptic bronchoscopic findings. The lesion originated in the right upper lobe and a tumor with smooth surface can be seen at the orifice of the right upper lobe bronchus.

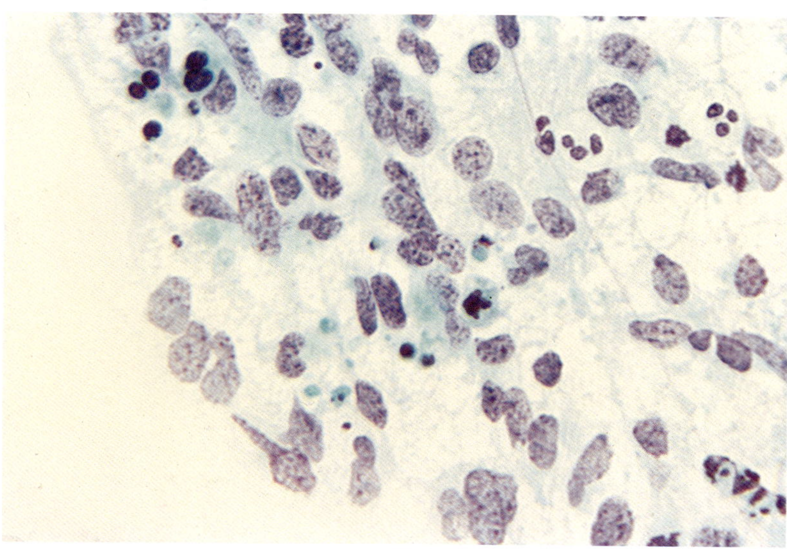

Fig. 125 Carcinoid in a transbronchial aspiration cytology specimen. Denuded nuclei are seen and the chromatin has increased in quantity. Intercellular adhesion of the cells is weak. The chromatin is finely granular and the nuclear membrane is regular and thin. The nuclear shape is polygonal. (X400, Pap.)

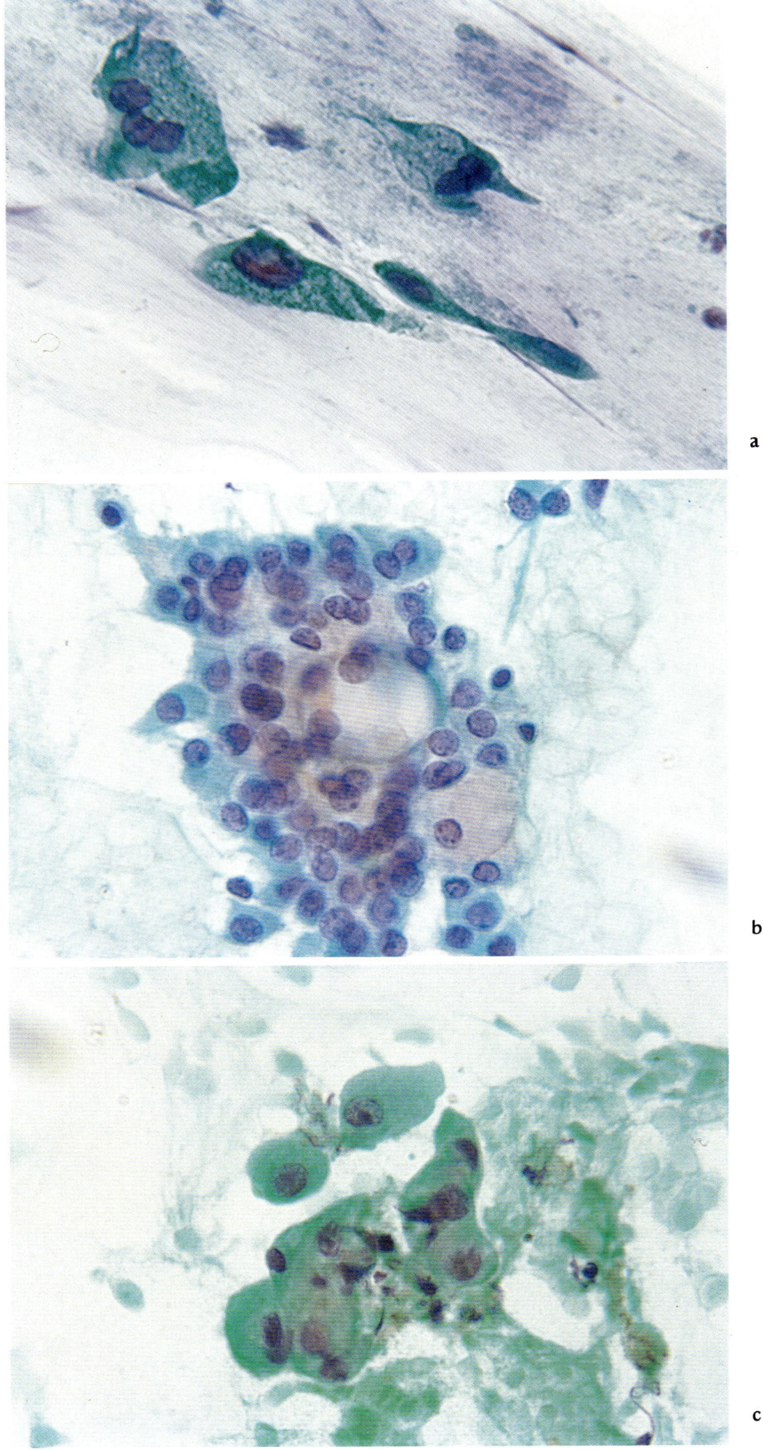

Fig. 126   See legend on page 120.

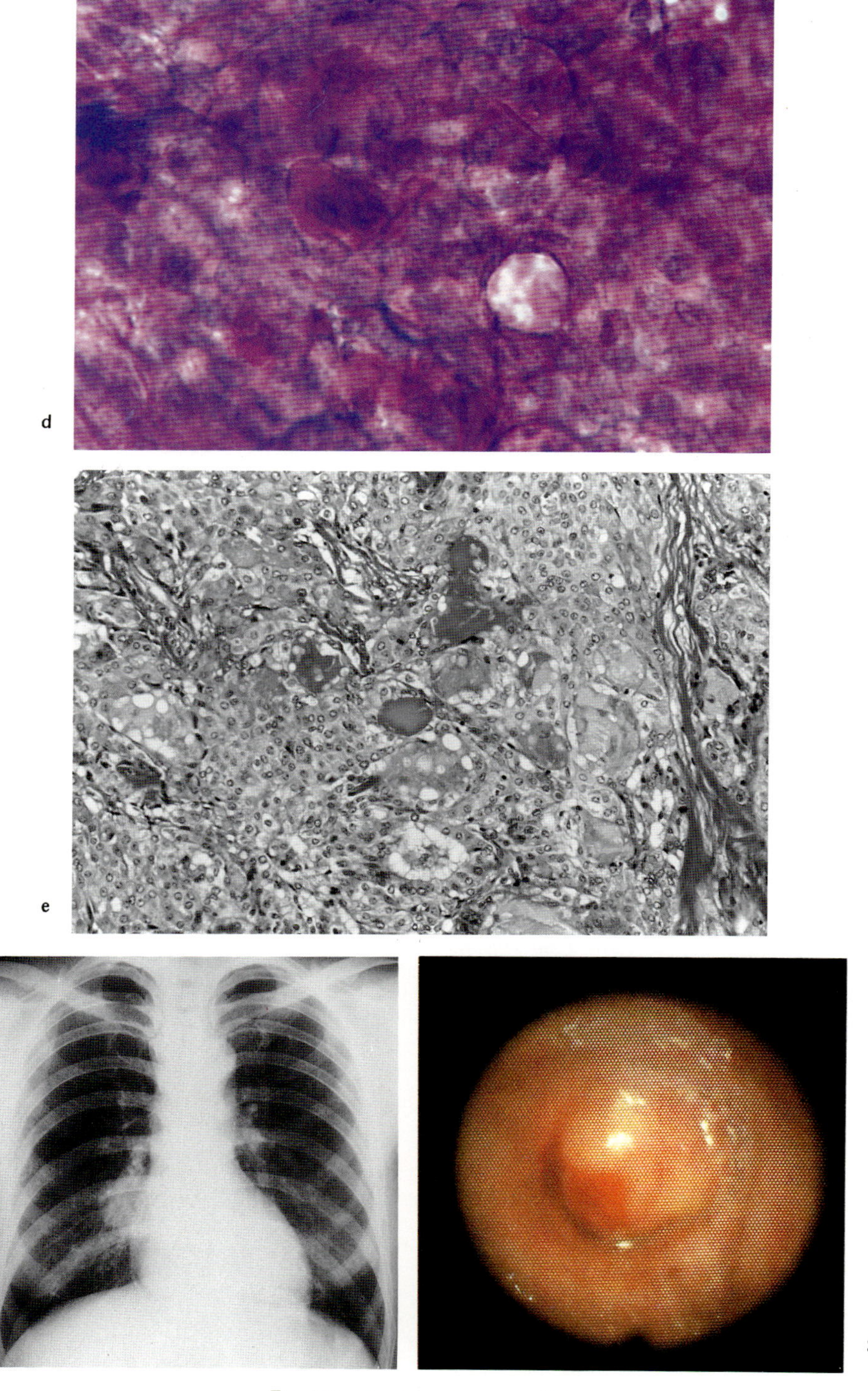

Fig. 126   See legend on page 120.

Clinical Findings: (Chest X-ray) This tumor develops usually in larger bronchi. Therefore tumor shadow can be seen in the hilar region with secondary changes and/or atelectasis. (Fiberoptic Bronchoscopy) Tumor is generally polypoid and is covered with normal epithelium. The surface is therefore smooth and glossy.

Sputum cytology specimens

The cells show degeneration as a result of exfoliation. Specimens contain cells resembling adenocarcinoma and atypical squamous metaplasia or squamous cell carcinoma (Matsuda et al., 1971). The former contain mucin vacuoles in their cytoplasm, whereas the cytoplasm of the latter strongly stains blue-green. The nuclear chromatin of both is increased in quantity and is finely to coarsely granular. The degree of morphologic atypia is usually low (Fig. 126a).

Brushing and needle cytology specimens

Because of the comparatively lesser degree of degeneration, brushing specimens show better stainability than do sputum specimens. The cells are slightly larger, and the very fine chromatin shows slight to moderate hyperchromasia. The cells resemble those of atypical squamous metaplasia and poorly differentiated squamous cell carcinoma and are mixed with cells containing mucin vacuoles in their cytoplasm (Fig. 126b-d).

Although it may be difficult to diagnose mucoepidermoid carcinoma on the basis of cytologic criteria alone, the diagnosis can usually be made by combining cytologic findings, fiberoptic bronchoscopic findings and clinical findings. The lesion typically appears endoscopically as a smooth-surfaced endobronchial polyp.

Fig. 126 Mucoepidermoid carcinoma.

(a) Sputum cytology specimen. Cells can be recognized in sputum after the tumor has invaded breaking through the bronchial mucosa or after bronchial biopsy. The cytoplasm is suggestive of squamous cell carcinoma because of its thickening and light green stain. Nuclei are frequently hyperchromatic and frequently have irregular borders. Mucin vacuoles can be recognized in the cytoplasm of the small cells shown in this figure. These are exfoliated cells in sputum and hence show a high degree of degeneration. (X400, Pap.)

(b) Brushing cytology specimen obtained after histologic biopsy. The cells display a low degree of atypia and at first glance resemble squamous metaplasia cells. The cytoplasm strongly stains light green. Some cells in the flat cluster possess much in their cytoplasm. There is little nuclear atypia. The nuclei are round with thin membranes and the nuclear chromatin does not show a significant increase in quantity. (X400, Pap.)

(c) Brushing cytology specimen. The degree of cellular atypia is greater than that of the cells in Figure (b), but is weaker than most invasive carcinoma cells. The cytoplasm stains a thick light green and the nuclear chromatin is increased in quantity, while the nuclear membrane is irregular. These findings resemble those of atypical squamous metaplastic cells. (X400, Pap.)

(d) Brushing cytology specimen. These are the PAS-stained findings. The mucin contained in the cytoplasm stains reddish purple. (X400, Pap.)

(e) Histologic findings. This tumor was of bronchial gland origin. Solid proliferation of a mixture of squamous cell carcinoma and mucus-producing tubules. (X200, H.E.)

(f) Chest X-ray findings of a 53-year-old woman. Tumor shadow with secondary change in the peripheral lung can be observed in the right lower lung field.

(g) Fiberoptic bronchoscopic findings. The tumor appeared as a smooth, glossy polyp covered by normal mucosa in the right lower lobe bronchus. In such cases, cells rarely appear in sputum.

ADENOID CYSTIC CARCINOMA

This type of tumor is thought to derive from the bronchial gland. It occurs most frequently in the trachea and large bronchi (Fig. 127b-d). It is a rare tumor, developing as a polyp with a certain degree of surface irregularity, although the surface is smooth. It grows invasively and shows distant metastasis in more than 50% of cases (Heilbrunn and Crosby, 1972). The endoscopic findings can usually be referred to when evaluating the cytologic findings.

Clinical Findings: (Chest X-ray) When the tumor originates in the trachea, no abnormal findings are observed in the chest X-ray film. Generally symptoms such as dyspnea appear. (Fiberoptic Bronchoscopy) The tumor surface is smooth and glossy because the tumor is covered by normal epithelium.

Sputum cytology specimens

This tumor is usually covered by normal bronchial mucosa; therefore, it is unusual for cells to be recognized in sputum specimens. When they do appear in such specimens, the cells are small, contain recognizable nucleoli and show a low degree of atypia. Mostly these are tightly clustered and tend to arrange around the lumen.

Brushing and needle cytology specimens

Ball-like and tight clumps of small, circular cells and cells containing mucin vacuoles can generally be seen. The degree of atypia is low. Nuclei are round and almost uniform in size. The amount of finely granular chromatin is not appreciably increased. Nucleoli are not recognized. Since this tumor is usually covered by normal mucosa, transbronchial aspiration (TBAC) is usually the most effective diagnostic approach, although brushing after histologic biopsy is also successful at times (Fig. 127b)

Fig. 127 Adenoid cystic carcinoma.
(a) Brushing cytology specimen. The materials were obtained by brushing cytology technique following histologic biopsy via the fiberoptic bronchoscope. The cells in ball-like clusters are small and rounded with little variation in size and show a low degree of atypia. The point that distinguishes them from basal cell hyperplastic cells, which they closely resemble, is the fact that basal hyperplasia does not appear in ball-like clusters. (X400, Pap.)
(b) Histologic findings. Islands of small polygonal cells with darkly staining nuclei are seen. Tubular lumens contain eosinophilic mucous. Variously sized cribriform lumens contain mucicarmine positive material. (X200, H.E.)
(c) Bronchographic findings. A tracheal tumor (arrow) is seen causing severe tracheal stenosis. Adenoid cystic carcinoma develops frequently in the trachea.
(d) Bronchoscopic findings. This is a smooth-surfaced, glossy tumor of bronchial gland origin that is seen to develop in the trachea and larger bronchi. Since it generally proliferates covered by normal bronchial mucosa, it rarely appears in sputum. This case originated in the trachea of a 60-year-old man who presented with dyspnea. Sputum cytology revealed no abnormal cells.

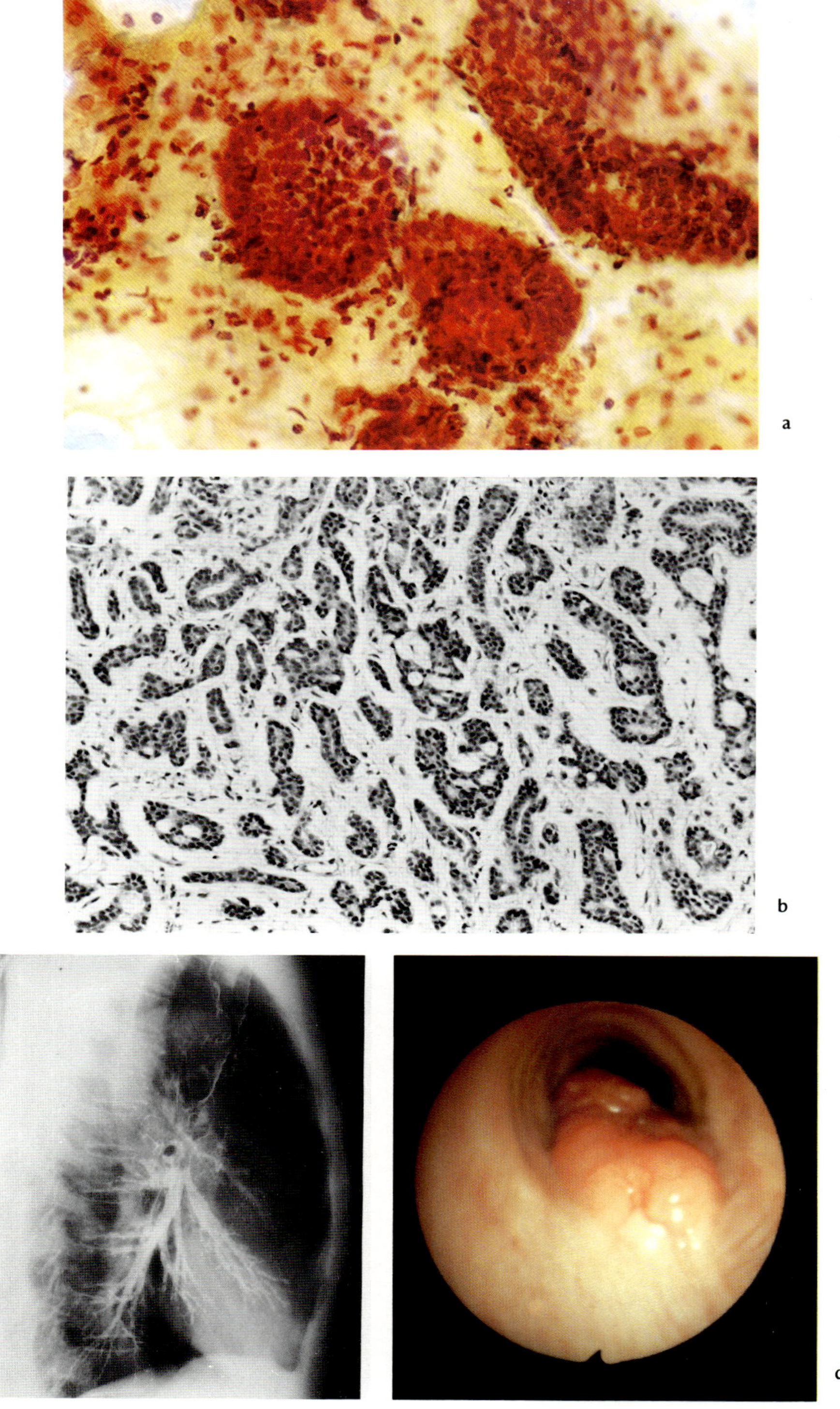

Fig. 127 See legend on page 121.

CARCINOSARCOMA

This tumor is also extremely rare. It is composed of a mixture of epithelial carcinoma and sarcomatous stroma. Cases of carcinosarcoma are combined with squamous cell carcinoma or adenocarcinoma (Fig. 128b-d). One theory holds that carcinomatous and sarcomatous components develop simultaneously (Takahashi, 1981) based on the fact that both components were found in metastatic foci (Chaudhuri, 1971; Diaconiţă, 1975), while another contends that the lesion represents sarcomatous changes of epithelial type malignant cells (Lane, 1957; Jenkins, 1968). The proliferation of this type of tumor is frequently characterized by its growth as a polyp in the bronchial lumen with no intramucosal invasion, and when this finding is recognized endoscopically, it can help the clinician to arrive at a correct diagnosis.

Clinical Findings: (Chest X-ray) This tumor proliferates rapidly as a polyp accompanied by obstruction of the bronchus. Therefore, atelectasis can frequently be seen on X-ray.
(Fiberoptic Bronchoscopy) The tumor is polypoid with a smooth surface and bleeds easily.

Sputum cytology specimens

In general, cancer cells composed of epithelial components are the most easily recognized; therefore, it is difficult to reach a histological diagnosis on the basis of the cytologic findings alone.

Brushing and needle cytology specimens

Brushing cytology yields specimens that contain both epithelial and nonepithelial materials. A cytologic diagnosis is possible when both elements are recognized. Brushing specimens contain slightly larger cells than do sputum specimens, the chromatin is very fine and the cells stain more distinctly in both elements. The epithelial components show each characteristic cellular features according to histologic type. However, the main epithelial component is that of squamous type. Nonepithelial components reveal spindle-like cells. The nuclei are round or oval with irregular and prominent nucleoli (Fig. 128a).

PULMONARY BLASTOMA

Pulmonary blastoma is a rare tumor which appears in peripheral locations. It consists of branching tubules or glands lined by a single layer of low columnar cells and immature mesenchymal cells, in which cartilagenous and osseous differentiation is seen. Since this histology resembles fetal lung (Barson et al., 1968; Karcioglu et al., 1974; Stackhouse et al., 1969), it was called embryoma by Barnard (1952). Cytologically pulmonary blastoma is characterized by co-existence of fibroblast-like spindly nuclei with delicate nuclear membrane and glandular epithelial cells, although cancer cells are rarely encountered.

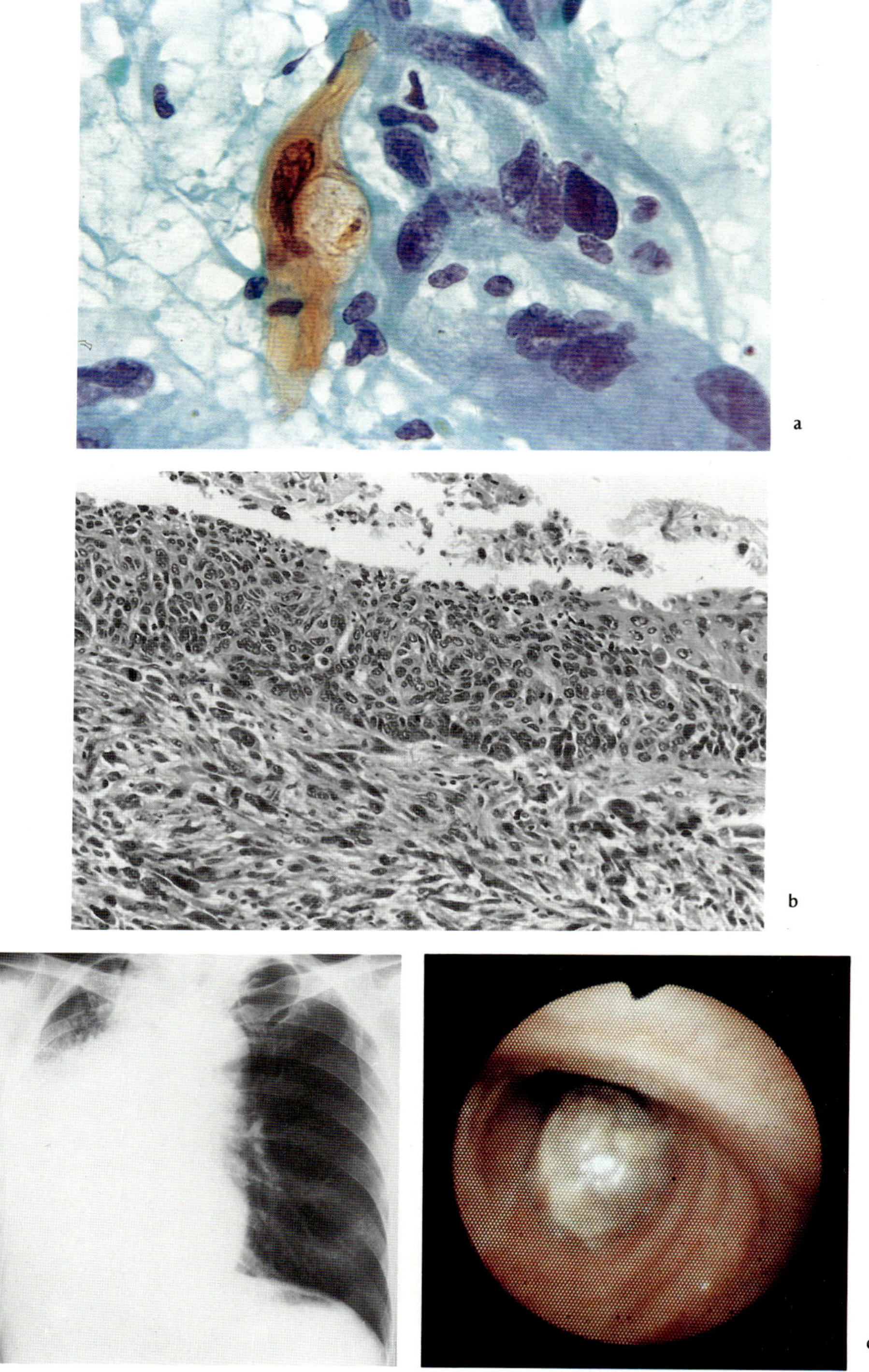

Fig. 128   See legend on opposite page.

Fig. 128 Carcinosarcoma.
(a) Brushing cytology specimen. The cytoplasm of the large, spindle-shaped cells stained light green and the elongated nuclei displayed increased chromatin, with one or more irregular nucleoli. These findings indicate malignant cells of non-epithelial origin, i.e. they suggest fibrosarcoma. Mixed with these cells are polygonal cells possessing keratinizing cytoplasm and strongly hyperchromatic nuclei, i.e. features of differentiated squamous cell carcinoma. In such cases in which two types of malignant cells can be recognized, carcinosarcoma should be suspected. The incidence of this type of tumor is extremely low. (X400, Pap.)
(b) Histologic findings. The histologic findings show squamous cell carcinoma in the superficial layer and fibrosarcoma in the submucosal layer. (X100, H.E.)
(c) Chest X-ray film of a 60-year-old man who presented with dyspnea. Atelectasis of the entire right lung is recognizable. Carcinosarcoma is frequently characterized by its growth as a polyp in the lumen of large airway, therefore atelectasis occurs frequently as the tumor proliferates.
(d) Fiberoptic bronchoscopic findings. Endoscopy revealed a polyp originating in the right main bronchus extending beyond the carina into the trachea. The surface was smooth and bled easily.

SARCOMA

Sarcoma of the lung is extremely rare and the incidence has been reported by Martini and coworkers (1971) to be less than 1% that of primary lung cancer. The following types of sarcomas of the lung have been reported: fibrosarcoma (Fig. 129) (Eskenasy, 1979), leiomyosarcoma, rhabdomyosarcoma, pleomorphic cell sarcoma, myxoliposarcoma, chondrosarcoma, angiosarcoma (Fig. 130), malignant lymphoma, neurosarcoma, etc. (Noehren and McKee, 1954; Hochberg and Crastnopol, 1956).

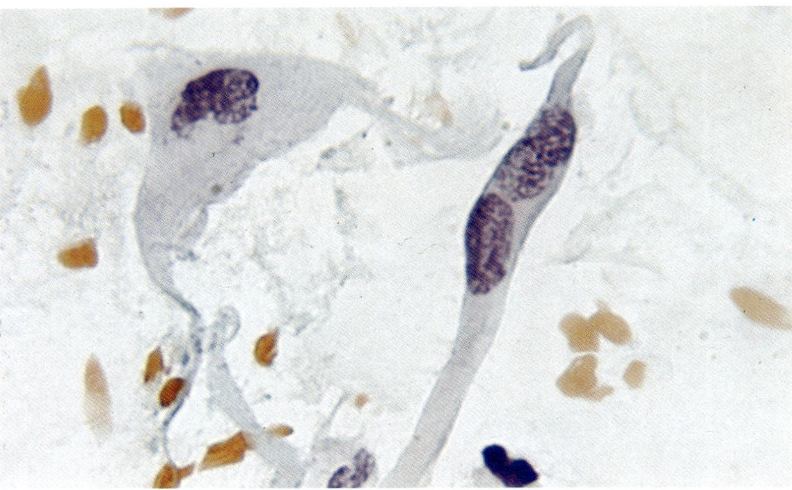

Fig. 129 Fibrosarcoma in a brushing cytology specimen. Cells with elongated cytoplasm and one or more irregular nuclei can be observed. Increased chromatin shows a reticular pattern. These findings indicate non-epithelial malignant cells. (X400, Pap.)

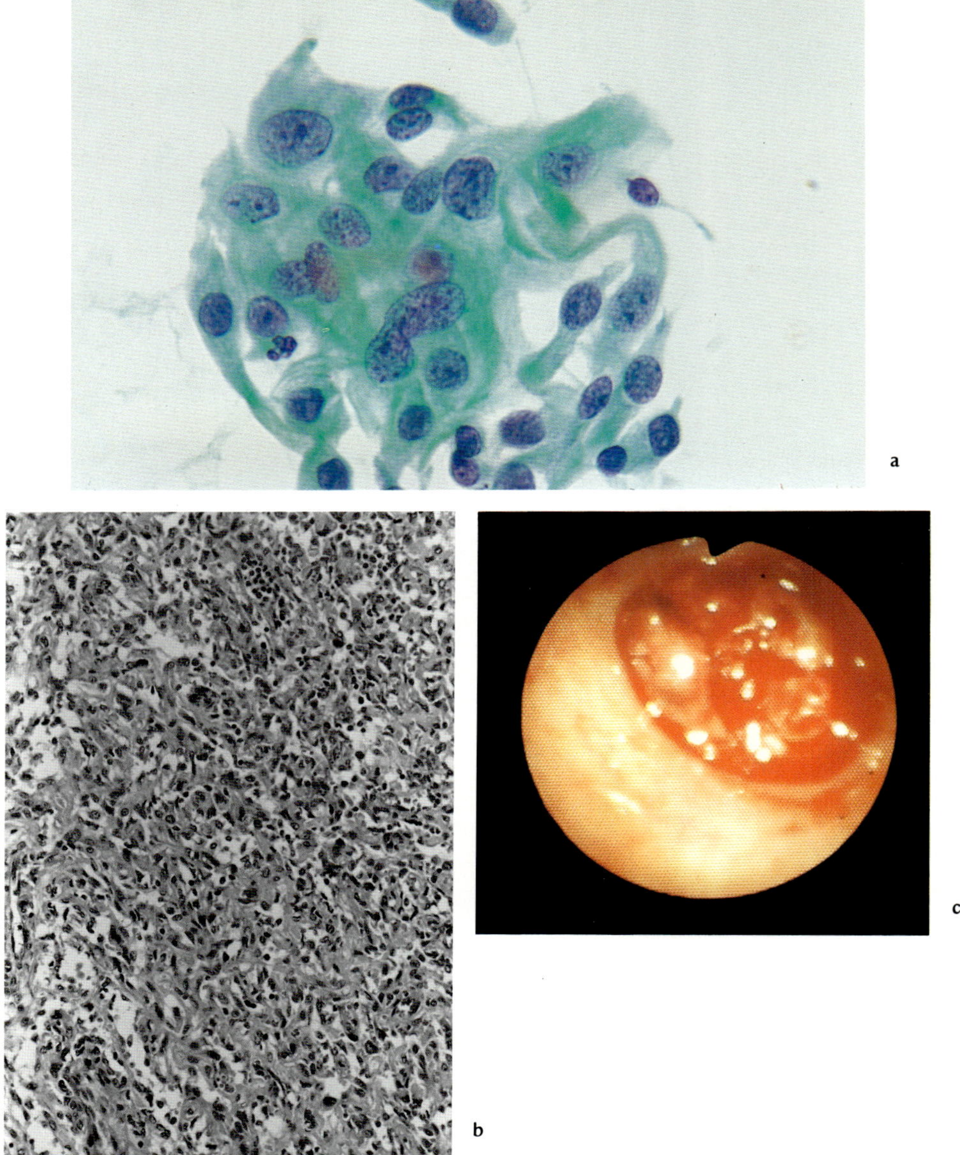

Fig. 130 Angiosarcoma.
(a)　Brushing cytology specimen. These tumor cells show poor adhesion and pleomorphism with occasional fiber-like appearance. The nuclei are round and almost identical in size. The cellular borders are difficult to distinguish, and the cytoplasm stains lightly. The nucleoli are prominent and the nuclear chromatin is not very hyperchromatic. (X400, Pap.)
(b)　Histologic findings. This tumor is composed of blood vessel endothelial cells. Numerous capillaries are observed throughout the entire specimen. (X200, H.E.)
(c)　Fiberoptic bronchoscopic findings. The left upper division bronchus is obstructed by a tumor with an irregular and bleeding surface. In general, this tumor can originate from malignant proliferation of vascular endothelium or epithelium.

METASTATIC LUNG TUMORS

Due to its nature, metastasis occurs easily in the lung (Abrams et al., 1950). Koss (1979) has reported that approximately 50% of tumors metastatic to the lungs may be diagnosed cytologically. Metastatic lesions frequently occur as tumor cell thrombi in narrow peripheral blood vessels; therefore, at an early stage, they usually do not connect directly with the bronchus and rarely appear in sputum specimens. Brushing under X-ray television guidance also sometimes fails to yield positive diagnostic materials, and therefore the most productive diagnostic methods are transbronchial aspiration and percutaneous needle cytology. As the lesion develops, it can become connected with bronchi, and cells begin to appear in the sputum.

Although infrequent, some lesions metastasize to the bronchial wall. If the tumor breaks through the bronchial membrane in cases of such endobronchial metastasis, cells can appear in the sputum. Metastasis to the bronchial wall most frequently occurs in cases of renal or rectal cancer. In such cases, it is difficult to determine the nature of the original primary tumor unless the patient's history is known (Figs. 131-139).

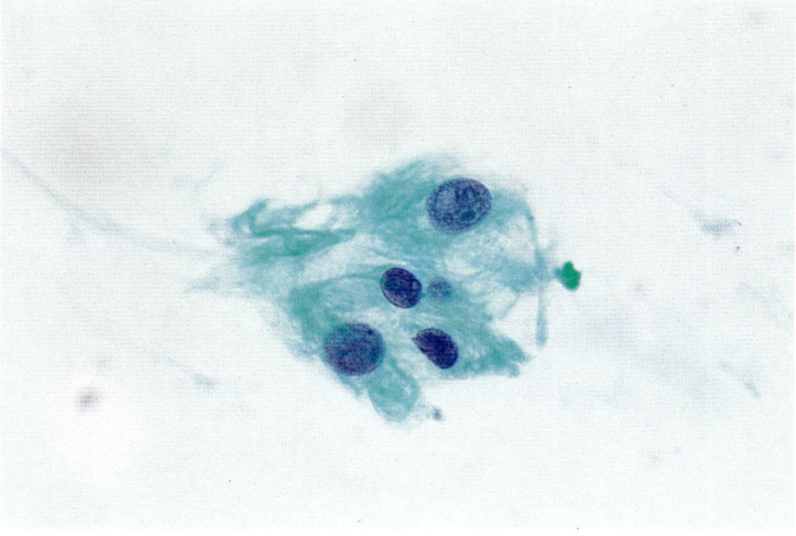

Fig. 131 Renal carcinoma in a brushing cytology specimen. Cells are large, polygonal in shape and with abundant cytoplasm. Cytoplasm is foamy. Nuclei are large with a prominent round nucleolus. This specimen was obtained by fiberoptic bronchoscopic brushing. (X400, Pap.)

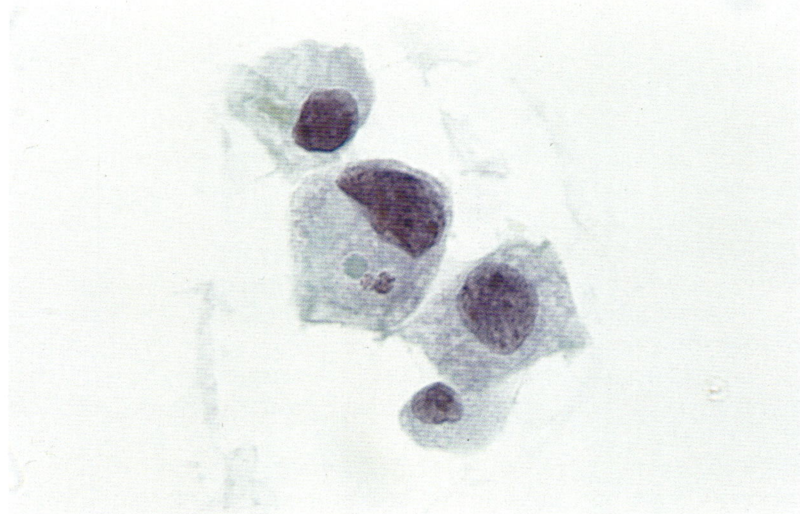

Fig. 132 Choriocarcinoma in a brushing cytology specimen. It is difficult to obtain cellular components from the lesion. It is characteristic that mostly hemorrhagic specimens are obtained. (X400, Pap.)

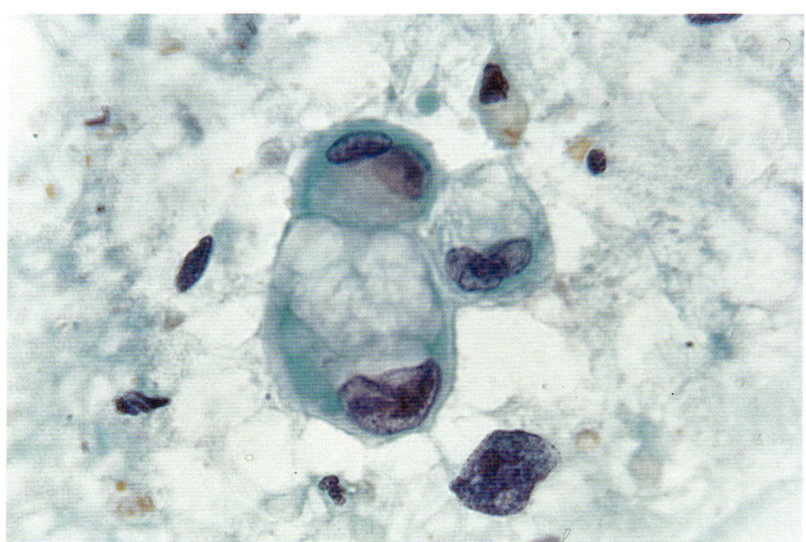

Fig. 133 Gastric cancer in a brushing cytology specimen. A basophilically stained cell cluster is observed. Generally hyperchromatism is not striking and multiple basophilic nucleoli are observed. (X400, Pap.)

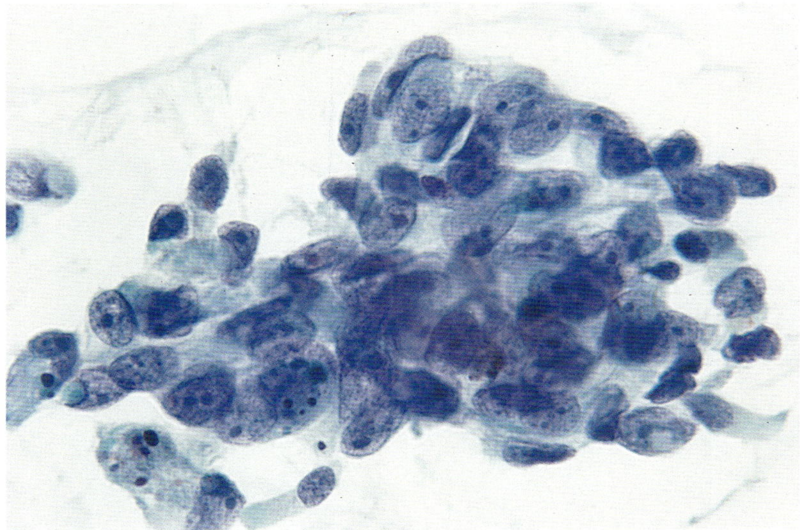

Fig. 134 Breast carcinoma in a brushing cytology specimen. Cell arrangement is papillary, and features indicate adenocarcinoma. (X400, Pap.)

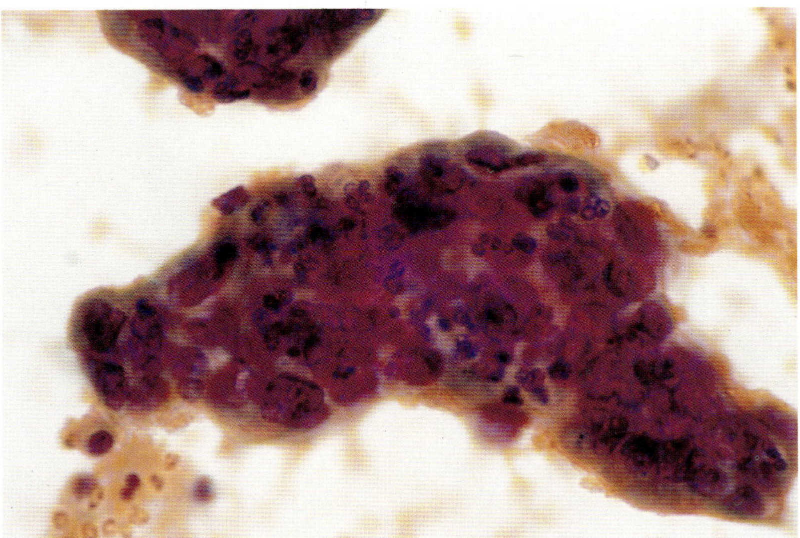

Fig. 135 Pancreas carcinoma in a brushing cytology specimen. A papillary cluster with eosinophilic cytoplasm is seen. Variation in nuclear size is recognized and some nuclei show hyperchromasia. (X400, Pap.)

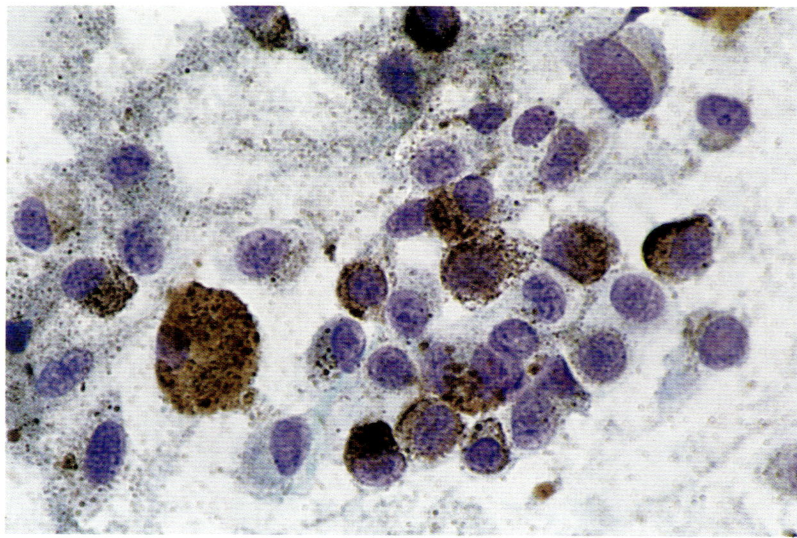

Fig. 136 Malignant melanoma in a sputum cytology specimen. The characteristic finding in the cytoplasm is marked brown pigmentation. The tumor cells and nuclei vary in size and have prominent nucleoli. (X400, Pap.)

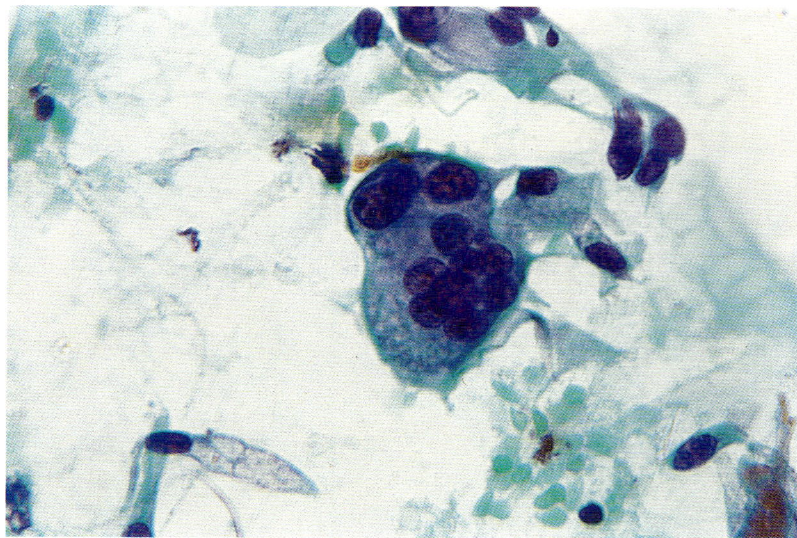

Fig. 137 Embryonic carcinoma in a brushing cytology specimen. Variation of cellular size is great. Cytoplasm stains basophilically. Nuclei show variation in size and are stained strongly by hematoxylin. Hyperchromatism is striking. (X400, Pap.)

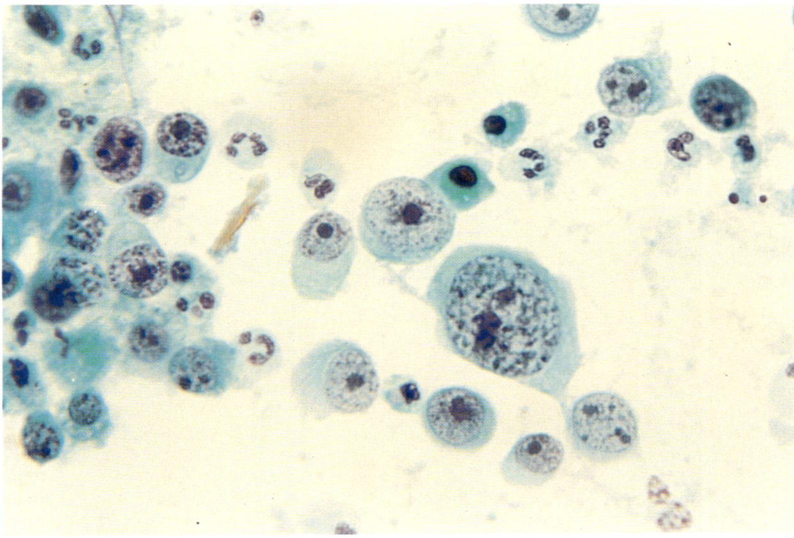

Fig. 138 Osteosarcoma in a brushing cytology specimen. The size of the polygonal cells varies remarkably. Intercellular adhesion is weak. Cytoplasm is foamy. The size of nuclei is variable and chromatin is coarse. Multinucleation and multinucleoli are often seen. (X400, Pap.)

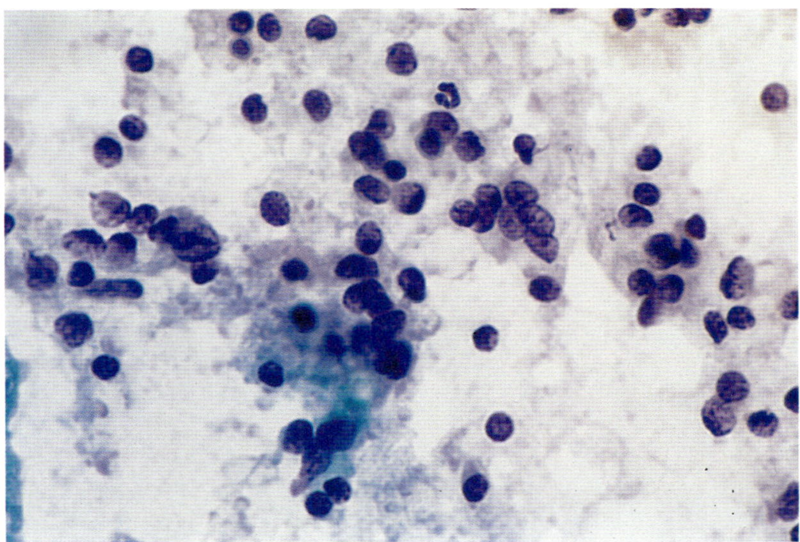

Fig. 139 Lymphosarcoma in a brushing cytology specimen. The cells are larger than lymphocytes but irregular in size with weak adhesion. Hyperchromasia is recognized and chromatin is coarsely granular. (X400, Pap.)

VII

Quantitative Cytochemistry

The morphologic diagnosis of cancer is based on a variety of factors related to nuclear atypia, such as increase in the nuclear-to-cytoplasmic ratio, variation in nuclear size, increase in the amount and irregular distribution of chromatin and increases in the amounts of nuclear deoxyribonucleic acid (DNA) (Sandritter et al., 1966; Wagner et al., 1967; Brandao, 1969; Böhm et al., 1971; Sachs et al., 1972a, 1972b; Sachs and Schäfer, 1973; Ludwig et al., 1973; Zetterberg and Esposti, 1976; Kato, 1977; Nasiell et al.,; 1978), ribonucleic acid (RNA) and protein resulting from the presence of the abnormal chromosomes of cancer cells. Therefore, measurements of nuclear DNA, RNA and protein can provide an objective method to evaluate the degree of malignancy and proliferation. Such an approach can also be employed to evaluate the response to anticancer therapy.

Cytochemical research on tumor cells began in 1940 with studies by Caspersson, who showed that large amounts of RNA exist in the nucleus and cytoplasm (Caspersson, 1979). In these decades, various attempts at measuring DNA and protein were made, and it was shown that the distribution pattern of DNA in some tumor cells is markedly different from that in normal cells. However, this finding has not yet been confirmed in all malignant diseases. It has also been recognized that there is a close interdependent relationship between nucleic acid and protein and that protein synthesis is deeply related to the cellular cycle. These findings have opened up a new path in the field of quantitative cytochemistry.

Methods in quantitative cytochemistry include examination of individual slides by microspectrophotometer and the flow method, in which floating cells are measured as they pass. The slide method is important for basic research because it allows identification of the individual cells. Meanwhile the speed that is required for this technique to be applied clinically means that the flow method is preferable for screening large numbers of specimens. However, it is probably better to consider the slide method and flow method as mutually complementary. Whereas DNA has been used as the primary material for such research, recent advances in instrumentation that permit simultaneous measurement of RNA and protein indicate that multiparameter evaluation of cells will yield even greater accuracy of cytochemical evaluation.

EVALUATION OF DEGREE OF MALIGNANCY OF LUNG CANCER BY MEASUREMENT OF DNA

DNA is one of the easiest cytochemical substances to measure. The relationship between the amount of DNA and the degree of malignancy is possible to evaluate if fresh cells from lung cancer lesions are obtained by brushing or aspiration techniques.

Figure 140 shows the histogram patterns of squamous cell carcinoma, small cell carcinoma and adenocarcinoma obtained by the needle aspiration cytology technique. The cells show a heteroploid distribution in modes above the tetraploid and their DNA distribution patterns are clearly different from normal cells.

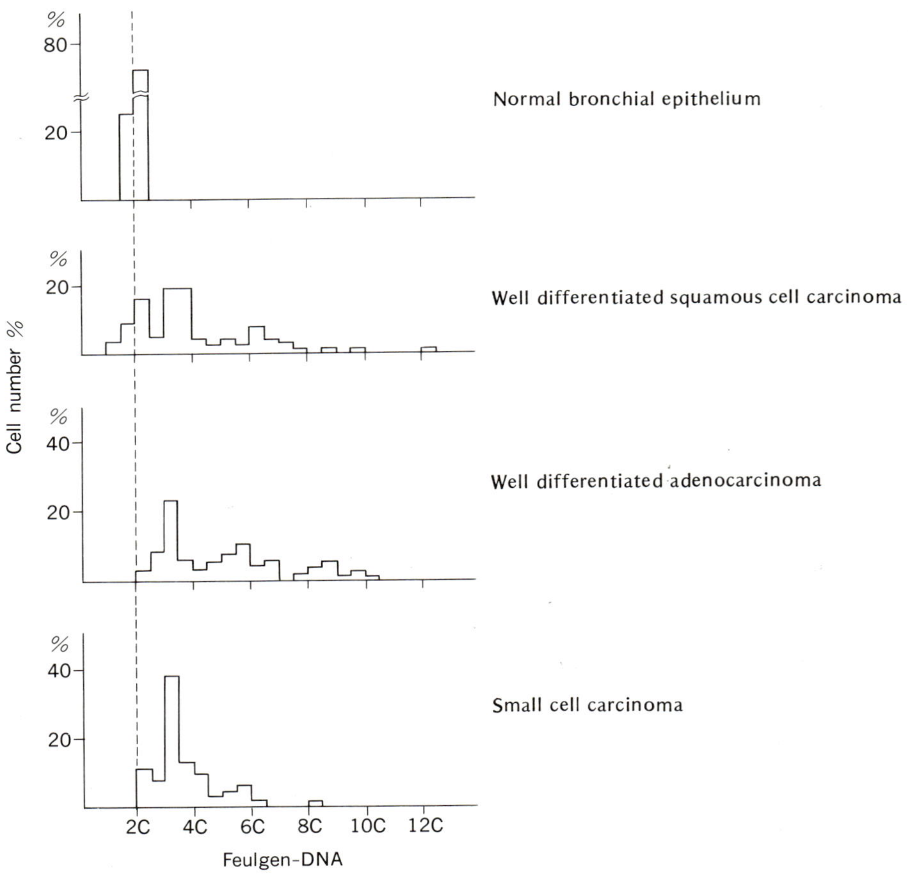

Fig. 140 Feulgen—DNA / Cell number (%)

CYTOCHEMICAL ANALYSIS OF CARCINOGENESES

Experiments involving the induction of lung cancer in dogs have demonstrated that intrabronchial injection of the carcinogen 20-methylcholanthrene results in the appearance of squamous cell metaplasia, followed by increasing degrees of atypia and culminating in the development of squamous cell carcinoma (Hayata et al., 1977; Kato et al., 1980b, 1982c; Konaka et al.,1982a, 1982b). As is shown in

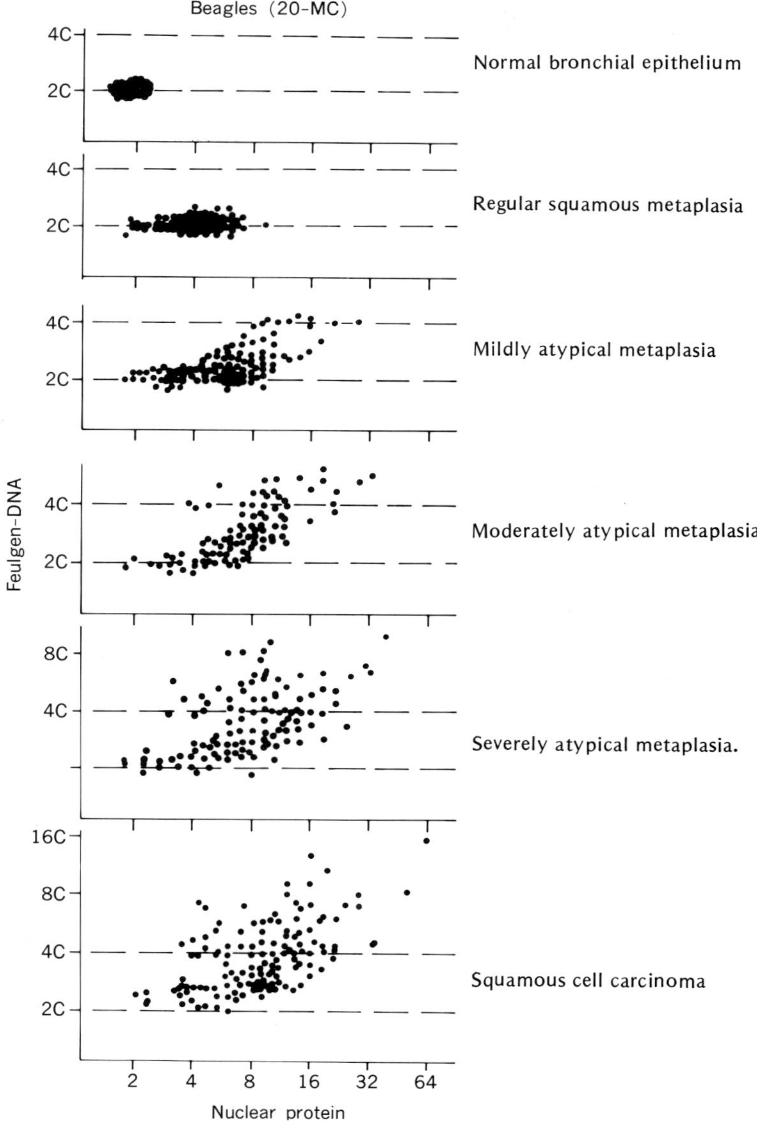

Fig. 141 Nuclear Protein / Feulgen-DNA
Previously published in Acta Histochem. Cytochem., 15: 779–797, 1982. (Konaka et al., 1982b.)

Figure 141, the DNA of mildly atypical squamous metaplastic cells is distributed from the diploid to the tetraploid modes and closely resembles the pattern obtained with normally growing cells. With moderate atypia, cells containing DNA in modes beyond the tetraploid region are recognized. Severely atypical squamous metaplastic cells show a heteroploid distribution resembling that of squamous cell carcinoma. Although there is no appreciable increase in the DNA compared to that of normal bronchial epithelial cells, a twofold to threefold increase in the amount of nuclear protein can be recognized in regular squamous metaplasia.

The relationship between DNA, nuclear protein and the cell phase of human lymphocytes is shown in Figure 142. Figure 141 shows that while the DNA

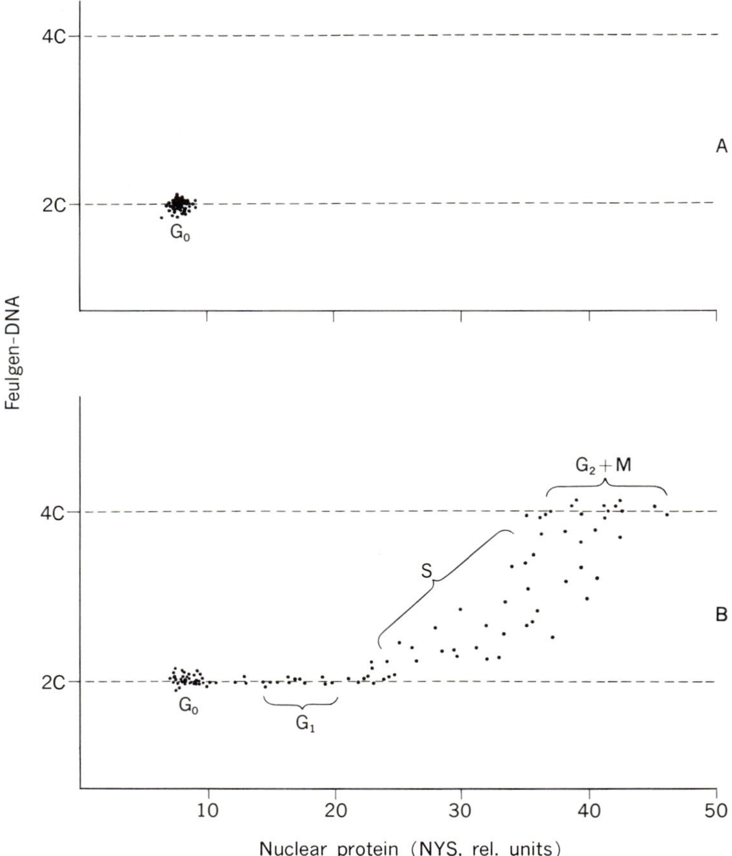

Fig. 142 Nuclear Protein / Feulgen-DNA
A: Normal lymphocytes (peripheral blood)
B: Cultured lymphocytes 72 hours after addition of phytohemagglutinin (PHA) to culture medium
GO: Cells outside the division cycle
G1: Presynthetic gap
S: DNA synthesis stage
G2: Postsynthetic gap
M: Mitotic division stage

pattern and protein observed in mildly and moderately atypical metaplastic cells
are not significantly different form those encountered in normal cells, the DNA
pattern and protein seen in severely atypical metaplastic cells resemble those
encountered in squamous cell carcinoma. The exact role of squamous metaplasia
in the development of squamous cell carcinoma has not been fully clarified, but
there does appear to be some interrelationship between these two conditions.

SENSITIVITY TESTS

The development of needle aspiration techniques has made it relatively simple to
harvest fresh cells from lesions (Azavedo et al., 1982). Short-term culture of the
small amount of cells thus obtained enables tests to be performed to evaluate the
effectiveness of therapeutic agents against cells of individual tumors. However, it
remains unknown whether tumor cells undergo cytochemical changes during the
culture process. Figure 143 shows that even at the first passage, one week after

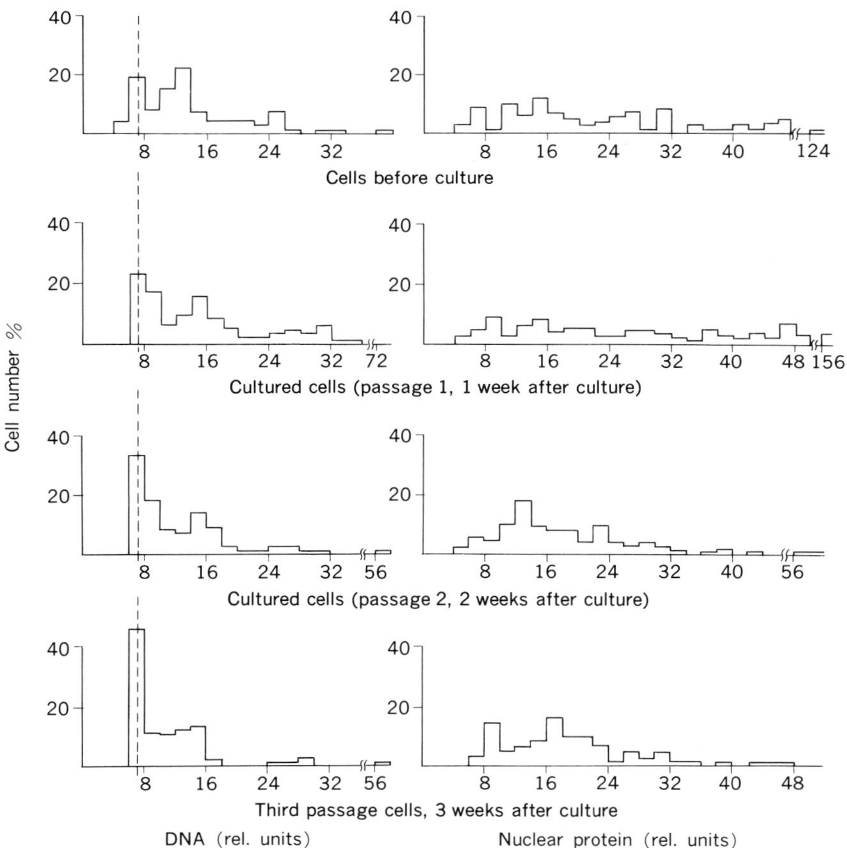

Fig. 143 Short-term culture of squamous cell carcinoma cells obtained by needle aspiration.

starting culture, changes can be seen in the DNA distribution pattern. This observation emphasizes the importance of establishing the most appropriate culture method for such procedures.

VIII

Flowchart of Cytologic Diagnosis

In the daily performance of clinical cytologic diagnosis, encounters with cells suspicious of malignancy are frequent. These belong to class II or III of Papanicolaou's classification. Their appearance can be the result of qualitative changes in materials from various kinds of pulmonary diseases and their treatment, borderline lesions of cancer and quantitative cancer cells from cancer lesions. The former consist of normal cells that have become abnormal due to the influence of certain factors and consist of abnormal columnar epithelial cells, basal cells, goblet cells, histiocytes, lymphocytes and atypical squamous metaplastic cells. The latter contain very few cancer cells and in terms of specimen collection, the danger of contamination by other specimens must be considered.

Cells imitating of the various histologic types of lung cancer are shown in Table 22. When such cells are encountered, it is difficult to make a correct diagnosis on the basis of the cellular appearance alone. Therefore it is necessary to take the clinical findings, roentgenological findings, endoscopic findings and histologic biopsy into account for an accurate definitive diagnosis.

At the authors' institution, clinical examination procedures are performed whenever suspicious cells are detected. If cancer is detected, treatment is performed and if a borderline lesion (severely atypical squamous metaplasia) is detected follow-up endoscopy is performed every three months. If no lesion can be detected follow-up sputum cytology is performed every three months (Fig. 144).

Table 22 Features of cells imitating cancer cells.

Squamous cell carcinoma	Adenocarcinoma	Large cell carcinoma	Small cell carcinoma
Squamous metaplasia with severe atypia	Hyperplasia of columnar cell	Atypical columnar cell	Atypical lymphocyte
Atypical columnar cell	Atypical goblet cell		Atypical histiocyte
Atypical basal cell hyperplasia	Atypical histiocyte		
Squamous cell carcinoma*	Adenocarcinoma*	Large cell carcinoma*	Small cell carcinoma*

* Insufficient numbers of cells.

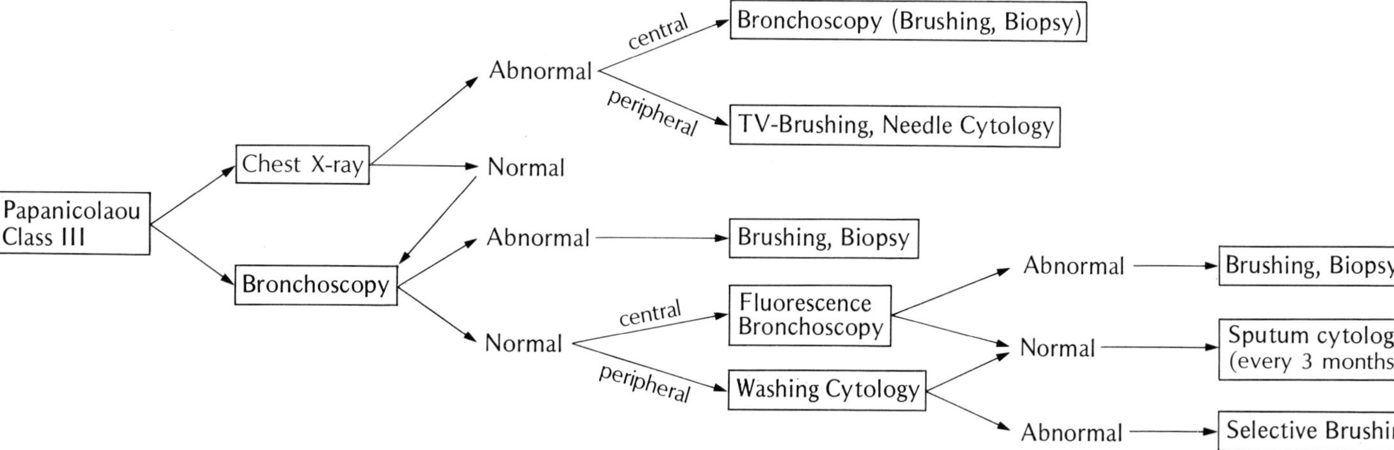

Fig. 144 Examination of a case with suspicious sputum cytology

Appendix
COMMON CHARACTERISTIC FINDINGS
OF LUNG CANCER
ACCORDING TO HISTOLOGIC TYPE

COMMON CHARACTERISTIC FINDINGS OF LUNG CANCER ACCORDING TO HISTOLOGIC TYPE

	Characteristic findings		
	Cytology	Fiberoptic bronchoscopy	Chest X-ray
Squamous cell carcinoma	Polygonal cells, Cannibalism *Pyknosis*	Irregular mucosa Exposed lesion in bronchial lumen	Hilar shadow, Secondary infiltrative shadow Atelectasis Cavity formation
Well diff.	Keratinization, *Cancer pearls* Bizarre shaped cells (fiber cells) Necrosis	Necrosis	
Poorly diff.	Thickening of basophilic cytoplasm		
Adenocarcinoma	Prominent round nucleolus Frothy basophilic cytoplasm	Central type: Swelling of bronchial mucosa due to submucosal proliferation Vascular engorgement Disappearance of mucosal folds Peripheral type: Usually not visible	Peripheral nodular shadow
Well diff.	Glandular papillary cluster Overlapping of cells Vacuolated cytoplasm		
Poorly diff.	Sheet-like arrangement Single cells		
Bronchioloalveolar cell carcinoma	Tightly packed clusters Cuboidal cells	Not visible	Multiple diffuse lesions
Small cell carcinoma	Small basophilic cells	Extramural compression due to lymph node involvement Widening of bifurcations	Lymphonode involvement shadows in the hilum and mediastinum without secondary changes
Oat cell type	*Pyknosis (India Ink)* Denuded nucleus		
Intermediate cell type	Variation of nuclear size More abundant cytoplasm than oat cell type		

Large cell carcinoma	Polygonal cell Single cell Prominent nucleoli Frothy cytoplasm	The same as those of adenocarcinoma	Tumor shadow in the hilum with or without secondary change
Giant cell type	Multinucleic giant cells		
Carcinoid	Moderate atypia Basophilic cells <u>Sheet-like arrangement</u> Resembles the intermediate cell type of small cell ca.	Polypoid tumor with smooth surface	Tumor shadow with secondary change and/or atelectasis
Mucoepidermoid carcinoma	Moderate atypia Resembles atypical squamous metaplastic cells Cytoplasmic vacuolation	Polypoid tumor with smooth surface	The same as carcinoid
Adenoid cystic carcinoma	Moderate atypia Ball-like cluster of small cells with round nuclei Mucin in the cluster	Frequently a polypoid tumor with a smooth surface in the trachea	No significant findings
Carcinosarcoma	Combination of epithelial and non-epithelial malignant cells	Polypoid proliferation with irregular surface Easy bleeding	Atelectasis

Italics : characteristic findings of sputum specimen
<u>Underlined</u> : characteristic findings of brushing or needle cytology specimen

REFERENCES

Abrams, H.L., Spiro, R. and Goldstein, N.: Metastases in carcinoma: Analysis of 1,000 autopsied cases. Cancer, 3: 74–85, 1950.

Adamson, Jr., J.S. and Bates, J.H.: Percutaneous needle biopsy of the lung. Arch. Int. Med., 119: 164–169, 1967.

Aronovitch, M., Chartier, J., Kahana, L.M. et al.: Needle biopsy as an aid to the precise diagnosis of intrathoracic disease. Canad. Med. Ass. J., 88: 120–127, 1963.

Azavedo, E., Tribukait, B. and Auer, G. et al.: Reproducibility of the cellular DNA-distribution patterns in multiple fine needle aspiration from human malignant tumors. Acta Pathol. Microbiol. Scand. Sect. A., 90: 79–83, 1982.

Ballin, A.: Ergebnisse pertrachealen Punktion. Zschr. Erkrank. Atmungsorgane, 148: 210–216, 1977. (in German with English abstract)

Barnard, W.G.: Embryoma of the lung. Thorax, 7: 299–301, 1952.

Barson, A.J., Jones, A.W. and Lodge, K.V.: Pulmonary blastoma. J. Clin. Pathol., 21: 480–485, 1968.

Bateson, E.M. and Abbott, E.K.: Mixed tumors of the lung or hamarto-chondromas: A review of the radiological appearances of cases published in the literature and a report of fifteen new cases. Clin. Radiol., 11: 232–247, 1960.

Bensch, K.G., Gordon, G.B. and Miller, L.R.: Studies on the bronchial counterpart of the Kultschitzky (Argentaffin) cell and innervation of bronchial glands. J. Ultrast. Res., 12: 668–686, 1965.

Bensch, K.G.: What is the function of the bronchial counterpart of the intestinal argentaffin (Kulchitsky) cell? Ann. Thorac. Surg., 14: 568–570, 1972.

Berger, R.L., Dargan, E.L. and Huang, B.L.: Dissemination of cancer cells by needle biopsy of the lung. J. Thorac. Cardiovasc. Surg., 63: 430–432, 1972.

Black, H. and Ackerman, L.V.: Importance of epidermoid carcinoma in situ in histogenesis of carcinoma of lung. Ann. Surg., 136: 44–55, 1952.

Böhm, N., Sprenger, E. and Sandritter, W.: Fluorescence Cytophotometric Feulgen-DNA Measurements of Benign and Malignant Human Tumors. Beitr. Path. Bd., 142: 210–220, 1971.

Brandão, H.J.S.: DNA Content in Epithelial Cells of Dysplasias of the Uterine Cervix. Histologic and Microspectrophotometric Observations. Acta Cytol., 13(4): 232–237, 1969.

Caspersson, T.: Quantitative tumor cytochemistry: G.H.A. Clowes Memorial Lecture. Cancer Res., 39: 2341–2355, 1979.

Chaudhuri, M.R.: Bronchial carcinosarcoma. J. Thorac. Cardiovasc. Surg., 61: 319–323, 1971.

Coleman, D.V.: The cytodiagnosis of human polyomavirus infection. Acta Cytol., 19: 93–96, 1975.

Craver, L.F. and Binkley, J.S.: Aspiration biopsy of tumors of the lung. J. Thorac. Surg., 8: 436–463, 1939.

Cutz, E. and Conen, P.E.: Ultrastructure and cytochemistry of Clara cells. Amer. J. Pathol., 62: 127–142, 1971.

Dahlgren, S.E.: Needle biopsy of intrapulmonary hamartoma. Scand. J. Respir. Dis., 47: 187–194, 1966.

Dahlgren, S.E.: Aspiration biopsy of intrathoracic tumors. Acta Pathol. Microbiol. Scand., 70: 566–576, 1967.

Diaconiţă, G.: Bronchopulmonary carcinosarcoma. Thorax, 30: 682–686, 1975.

Doiron, D.R., Profio, E., Vincent, R.G. et al.: Fluorescence bronchoscopy for detection of lung cancer. Chest, 76: 27–32, 1979.

Dutra, F.R. and Geraci, C.L.: Needle biopsy of the lung. J.A.M.A., 155: 21–24, 1954.

Endo, M. et al.: Observation of esophageal mucosa by dye scattering method. Progress of Digestive Endoscopy. 1: 34, 1972 (in Japanese).

Eskenasy, A.: Primary lung sarcomas: A histopathologic study of 118 cases. Morphol. Embryol. Physiol., 25: 27–38, 1979.

Franzén, S. and Zajicek, J.: Aspiration biopsy in diagnosis of palpable lesions of the breast. Critical review of 3,479 consecutive biopsies. Acta radiol., Stockh. 7: 241–262, 1968.

Gledhill, E.Y., Spriggs, J.B. and Binford, C.H.: Needle aspiration in the diagnosis of lung carcinoma: Report of experience with 75 aspirations. Amer. J. Clin. Pathol., 19: 235–242, 1949.

Grunze, H.: Derzeitiger Stand der Zytodiagnostik bei Erkrankungen des Thorax. Dtsch. Med. Wschr., 91: 1476–1483, 1966.

Hattori, S., Matsuda, M., Sugiyama, T. et al: Cytologic diagnosis of early lung cancer: Brushing method under X-ray television fluoroscopy. Dis. Chest, 45: 129–142, 1964.

Hattori, S., Matsuda, M., Sugiyama, T. et al.: Cytologic diagnosis of early lung cancer: An improved TV-brushing method and a review of negative results. Dis. Chest, 48: 123–129, 1965.

Hattori, S.: Cytologic diagnosis of peripheral lung lesions. In: Compendium on Diagnostic Cytology, Tutorials of Cytology, Chicago, 1979. pp. 349–355.

Hayata, Y., Kato, H., Chow, M.C. et al.: Studies of the carcinogenetic process in experimental squamous cell carcinoma in canine lungs. Jap. J. Thorac. Dis., 15: 759–768, 1977. (in Japanese with English abstract)

Hayata, Y. and Kato, H.: Cytology of the respiratory tract. Medicina, 16: 1998–2001, 1979. (in Japanese)

Hayata, Y., Oho, K., Ichiba, M. et al.: Percutaneous pulmonary puncture for cytologic diagnosis: Its diagnostic value for small peripheral pulmonary carcinoma. Acta Cytol., 17: 469–475, 1973.

Hayata, Y., Kato, H., Konaka, C. et al.: Fiberoptic bronchoscopic laser photoradiation for tumor localization in lung cancer. Chest, 82, 1, 10–14, 1982a.

Hayata, Y., Kato, H., Ono, J. et al.: Fluorescence fiberopitic bronchoscopy in the diagnosis of early stage lung cancer. In: Band, P.R. (ed.) Early Detection and Localization of Lung Tumors in High Risk Groups, Recent Results in Cancer Research, No. 82, Springer-Verlag, Berlin, Heidelberg, New York, 1982b. pp. 121–130.

Heilbrunn, A. and Crosby, I.K.: Adenocystic carcinoma and mucoepidermoid carcinoma of the tracheobronchial tree. Chest, 61: 145–149, 1972.

Hiddink, R.H.J. and Lopes Cardozo, P.: Aspiration cytology. Proceedings of the Sixth International Congress of Cytology. Tokyo, 1977. pp. 52.

Hochberg, L.A. and Crastnopol, P.: Primary sarcoma of the bronchus. Amer. Surg., 73: 74–98, 1956.

Ichiba, M., Tsuji, K., Takakura, N. et al.: A case of needle tract implantation as a result of needle biopsy for lung cancer. J. Jap. Lung Cancer Soc., 15: 337–342, 1975. (in Japanese with English abstract)

Ide, G., Hayashi, Y., Ogata, G. et al.: Histopathological and histochemical study on mucosal surface of the airway in pulmonary carcinoma cases. Igaku-no-Ayumi (Progress of Medicine), 59: 465–469, 1966. (in Japanese)

Ikeda, S.: Atlas of Flexible Bronchofiberscopy. Igaku-shoin, Tokyo, 1974.

Jacques, J. and Currie, W.: Bronchiolo-alveolar carcinoma: A Clara cell tumor? Cancer, 40: 2171–2180, 1977.

Jenkins, B.J.: Carcinosarcoma of the lung: Report of a case and review of the literature. J. Thorac. Cardiovasc. Surg., 55: 657–662, 1968.

Johnsson, K.A. and Schnürer, L.B.: Resultat av punktionscytologi vid utredning av lunginfiltrat. Nord. Med., 86: 1288, 1971. (in Swedish)

Johnston, W.W. and Frable, W.J.: The cytopathology of the respiratory tract: A review. Amer. J. Pathol., 84: 372–414, 1976.

Karcioglu, Z.A. and Someren, A.O.: Pulmonary blastoma: A case report and review of the literature. Am. J. Clin. Pathol., 61: 287–295, 1974.

Kato, H., Hayata, Y., Nasiell, M. et al.: The process of the development of pulmonary squamous cell carcinoma and cytophotometric DNA analysis: In respect of squamous cell metaplasia of bronchial epithelium, Carcinoma in situ and keratinized squamous cell carcinoma. Lung Cancer, 17: 267–279, 1977. (in Japanese with English abstract)

Kato, H., Ono, J., Niizuma, M. et al.: Transbronchofiberscopic aspiration biopsy using a special catheter. Jap. J. Thorac. Dis., 16: 774–780, 1978a. (in Japanese with English abstract)

Kato, H., Hayata, Y., Oho, K. et al.: Bronchofiberscopical findings of bronchial atypical squamous cell metaplasia, carcinoma in situ and early stage lung cancer. In: Proceedings of the World Congress on Bronchoscopy, July 9–12, 1978b, Tokyo. pp. 73–78.

Kato, H., Seo, Y., Ono, J. et al.: Squamous metaplasia and squamous cell carcinoma of the lung. Chiryo (Journal of Therapy), 61: 1325–1332, 1979. (in Japanese)

Kato, H., Kawate, N., Matsushima, Y. et al.: Percutaneous needle (cytological) biopsy of the lung. Jap. J. Clin. Pathol., Suppl. 41: 95–109, 1980a. (in Japanese)

Kato, H., Saito, T., Ono, J. et al.: Carcinogenetic process of central type squamous cell carcinoma in dogs and clinical application. Lung Cancer, 20: 53–62, 1980b. (in Japanese)

Kato, H., Hayashi, T., Konaka, C. et al.: Squamous metaplasia and squamous cell carcinoma. J. Jap. Soc. Clin. Cytol., 19 (4-Suppl.): 29–34, 1980c. (in Japanese)

Kato, H., Konaka, C., Ono, J. et al.: Cancer localization by detection of fluorescence by means of HpD administration and krypton ion laser photoradiation in canine lung cancer. Lung Cancer, 21: 439–445, 1981a. (in Japanese with English abstract)

Kato, K., Nishimiya, K., Lei, J. et al.: Transbronchial needle aspiration biopsy via the fiberoptic bronchoscope. In: Nakhosteen, J.A. and Maassen, W. (eds.) Bronchology: Research, Diagnostic, and Therapeutic Aspects, Martinus Nijhoff Publishers, The Hague, 1981b. pp. 307–309.

Kato, H., Hino, H., Nishimiya, K. et al.: Cytology and biopsy of lung cancer. Jap. J. Soc. Cancer Ther., 16: 490–491, 1981c. (in Japanese)

Kato, H.: Sputum cytology diagnosis. In: Hayata, Y. (ed.) Lung Cancer Diagnosis, Igaku-Shoin, Tokyo and New York, 1982. pp. 85–101.

Kato, H. and Konaka, C.: Morphology of fresh cytology specimens in pulmonary tumors. In: Hayata, Y. (ed.) Lung Cancer Diagnosis, Igaku-Shoin, Tokyo and New York, 1982. pp. 139–153.

Kato, H. and Ono, J.: Transbronchial aspiration cytology (TBAC). In Hayata, Y. (ed.) Lung Cancer Diagnosis, Igaku-Shoin, Tokyo and New York, 1982. pp. 127–131.

Kato, H. et al.: Lung cancer survey using television programs. Lung Cancer, (in press) 1982a.

Kato, H., Konaka, C., Sawa, H. et al.: Diagnosis and treatment of early lung cancer. Geka Chiryo (Surgical

Treatment), 24: 284—292, 1982b. (in Japanese)

Kato, H., Konaka, C., Hayata, Y. et al.: Lung cancer histogenesis following in vivo bronchial infections of 20-methylcholanthrene in dogs. In: Band, P.R. (ed.) Early Detection and Localization of Lung Tumors in High Risk Groups, Recent Results in Cancer Research, No. 82, Springer-Verlag, Berlin, Heidelberg, New York, 1982c. pp. 69—86.

Kawai, N. and Katsuki, H.: Relationship between tuberculosis and cancer of the lung. Kekkaku (Tuberculosis), 31 (Suppl.): 1—28, 1956. (in Japanese)

King, E.G., Bachynski, J.E. and Mielke, B.: Percutaneous trephine lung biopsy. Chest., 70: 212—216, 1976.

Kinsey, J.H., Cortese, D.A. and Sanderson, D.R.: Detection of hematoporphyrin fluorescence during fiberoptic bronchoscopy to localize early bronchogenic carcinoma. Mayo Clin. Proc., 53: 594—600, 1978.

Kobayashi, N., Okita, T., Hanzawa, S. et al.: A method for experimental injection of bronchogenic carcinoma in subcutaneously implanted bronchial autograft in dogs. J. Thorac. Cardiovasc. Surg., 75: 434—442, 1978.

Konaka, C., Auer, G., Nasiell, M. et al.: Pathogenesis of squamous bronchial carcinoma in 20-methylcholanthrene-treated beagle dogs. Analyt. Quant. Cytol., 4: 61—71, 1982a.

Konaka, C., Auer, G., Nasiell, M. et al.: Sequential cytomorphological and cytochemical changes during development of bronchial carcinoma in beagle dogs exposed to 20-methylcholanthrene. Acta Histochem. Cytochem., 15: 779—797, 1982b.

Koss, L.G.: Diagnostic Cytology and Its Histopathologic Bases, 3rd ed., J.B. Lippincott Company, Philadelphia, 1979.

Lane, N.: Pseudosarcoma (polypoid sarcoma-like masses) associated with squamous-cell carcinoma of the mouth, fauces, and larynx: Report of ten cases. Cancer, 10: 19—41, 1957.

Lauby, V.W., Burnett, W.E., Rosemond, G.P. et al.: Value and risk of biopsy of pulmonary lesions by needle aspiration, J. Thorac. Cardiovasc. Surg., 49: 159—172, 1965.

Leyden, O.O.: Über infektiöse Pneumonie. Dtsch. Med. Wschr., 9: 52—54, 1883.

Ludwig, A.S., Okazaki, T., Richart, R.M. and Lattes, R.: Nuclear DNA Content of Lobular Carcinoma in situ of the Breast. Cancer, 31: 1553—1560, 1973.

Marchesani, W.: Über den primären Bronchialkrebs. Frankfurt. Z. Path., 30: 158—190, 1924.

Marchok, A.C., Cone, M.V. and Nettesheim, P.: Induction Squamous Metaplasia (Vitamin A Deficiency) and Hypersecretory Activity in Tracheal Organ Cultures. 33(4): 451—460, 1975.

Martin, H.E. and Ellis, E.B.: Biopsy by needle puncture and aspiration. Ann, Surg., 92: 169—181, 1930.

Martini, N., Hajdu, S.I. and Beattie, Jr., E.J.: Primary sarcoma of the lung. J. Thorac. Cardiovasc. Surg., 61: 33—38, 1971.

Matsuda, M., Tateishi, R., Horai, T. et al.: Mucoepidermoid carcinoma of the bronchus. Lung Cancer, 11: 291—307, 1971. (in Japanese with English abstract)

Meckstroth, C.V., Davidson, H.B. and Kress, G.O.: Muco-epidermoid tumor of the bronchus. Dis. Chest, 40: 652—656, 1961.

Melamed, M.R., Zaman, M.B., Flehinger, B.J. et al.: Radiologically occult in situ and incipient invasive epidermoid lung cancer: Detection by sputum cytology in a survey of asymptomatic cigarette smokers. Amer. J. Surg. Pathol., 1: 5—16, 1977.

Ménétrier, P.: Cancer primitif du poumon. Bull. Soc. Anat., 11: 643—647, 1886.

Meyer, J.E., Ferrucci, Jr., J.T. and Janower, M.L.: Fatal complications of percutaneous lung biopsy. Radiology, 96: 47—48, 1970.

Naib, Z.M., Stewart, J.A., Dowdle, W.R. et al.: Cytological features of viral respiratory tract infections. Acta Cytol., 12: 162—171, 1968.

Nakajima, H., Hayata, Y., Hayashi, N. et al.: Experimental lung cancer produced in dogs by intrabronchial application of 20-methylcholanthrene: Technique and characteristics of induced tumors. Lung Cancer, 15: 53—60, 1975. (in Japanese with English abstract)

Nasiell, M.: The general appearance of the bronchial epithelium in bronchial carcinoma: A histopathological study with some cytological viewpoints. Acta Cytol., 7: 97—106, 1963.

Nasiell, M.: Metaplasia and atypical metaplasia in the bronchial epithelium: A histopathologic and cytopathologic study. Acta Cytol., 10: 421—427, 1966.

Nasiell, M.: Comparative histological and sputumcytological studies of the bronchial epithelium in inflammatory and neoplastic lung disease. Acta Path. Microbiol. Scand., 72: 501—518, 1968.

Nasiell, M., Roger, V., Nasiell, K. et al.: Cytologic findings indicating pulmonary tuberculosis: I. The diagnostic significance of epithelioid cells and Langhans' giant cells found in sputum or bronchial secretions. Acta Cytol., 16: 146—151, 1972.

Nasiell, M., Kato, H., Auer, G. et al.: Cytomorphological grading and Feulgen DNA analysis of metaplastic and neoplastic bronchial cells. Cancer, 41: 1511—1521, 1978.

Nasiell, M.: Cytology of benign changes and carcinoma in situ of the lung. In: Compendium on Diagnostic Cytology, 4th ed., Tutorials of Cytology, Chicago, 1979. pp. 315—329.

Niskanen, K.O.: Observations on metaplasia of the bronchial epithelium and its relation to carcinoma of the lung: Pathoanatomical and experimental researches. (Transl. by E. Harbén.) Acta Path. Microbiol. Scand. 80 (Suppl.): 1—80, 1949.

Noehren, T.H. and McKee, F.: Sarcoma of the lung. Dis. Chest, 25: 663–678, 1954.

Nordenström, B. and Dahlgren, N.: Transthoracic Needle Biopsy. Almqvist & Wiksell, Stockholm, 1966.

Nordenström, B.: New instruments for biopsy. Radiology, 117: 474–475, 1975.

Ochsner, A., DeBakey, M. and Dixon, J.L.: Primary cancer of the lung. J. A. M. A., 135: 321–327, 1947.

Oiwa, T., Okamoto, T., Yarita, Y. et al.: A case of pneumocystis carinii pneumonia. Nippon Kyobu Rinsho (Japanese Journal of Clinical Chest Disease), 39: 900–905, 1980. (in Japanese with English abstract)

Okada, Y.: Lung Cancer, Igaku-Shoin Ltd., Tokyo, 1972. (in Japanese)

Okamoto, T., Matsumura, K., Hanzawa, S. et al.: Percutaneous needle biopsy of the lung: Complications and indications. Jap. J. Thorac. Dis., 12: 676–682, 1974. (in Japanese with English abstract)

Oldham, Jr., H.N.: Benign tumors of the lung and bronchus. Surg. Clin. North Amer., 60: 825–834, 1980.

Ono, J.: Evaluation of therapeutic effectiveness in advance lung cancer by Feulgen-DNA quantitative analysis of cell nucleic. Lung Cancer, 21: 127–141, 1981. (in Japanese with English abstract)

Ono, J., Auer, G., Kato, H. et al.: Simultaneous analysis of cytomorphological, cytometrical and cytochemical cellular alterations during induction of bronchogenic carcinoma in dog. Cancer Res., (in press).

Ono, J. et al.: (1982) unpublished data

Oota, K.: A comment to Miyakawa, M. and Shibata, I.: Histopathologic studies on metaplasia of mucous epithelium from viewpoint of carcinogenesis. Gann., 46: 284–287, 1955.

Papanicolaou, G.N.: A new procedure for staining vaginal smears, Science, 95: 438–439, 1942.

Papanicolaou, G.N.: Degenerative changes in ciliated cells exfoliating from the bronchial epithelium as a cytologic criterion in the diagnosis of diseases of the lung. N. Y. J. Med., 56: 2647–2650, 1956.

Papanicolaou, G.N., Bridges, E.L. and Railey, C.: Degeneration of the ciliated cells of the bronchial epithelium (ciliocytophthoria) in its relation to pulmonary disease. Amer. Rev. Resp. Dis., 83: 641–659, 1961.

Pearson, F.G., Thompson, D.W. and Band, P.R.: The Sputum Cytology Program for Uranium Workers, Elliot Lake Centre d'Elliot Lake, Ontario, Canada.

Pichlmaier, H., Erpenbeck, R. and Finsterer, H.: Erweiterung der Lungendiagnostik durch transtrachelale und transbronchiale Lungenpunktion und gezielte segmentale Absaugung. Thoraxchirurgie Vaskläre Chirurgie, 18: 410–416, 1970.

Profio, A.E. and Doiron, D.R.: A feasibility study of the use of fluorescence bronchoscopy for localization of small lung tumors. Phys. Med. Biol., 22: 949–957, 1977.

Ramzy, I.: Pulmonary hamartomas: Cytologic appearances of fine needle aspiration biopsy. Acta Cytol., 20: 15–19, 1976.

Rhodin, J.A.G.: Ultrastucture and function of the human tracheal mucosa. Amer. Rev. Resp. Dis., 93 (Suppl.): 1–15, 1966.

Roger, V., Nasiell, M., Linden, M. et al.: Cytologic differential diagnosis of bronchiolo-alveolar carcinoma and bronchogenic adenocarcinoma. Acta Cytol., 20: 303–307, 1976.

Saccomanno, G., Saunders, R.P., Ellis, H. et al.: Concentration of carcinoma or atypical cells in sputum. Acta Cytol., 7: 305–310, 1963.

Saccomanno, G., Archer, V.E., Auerbach, O. et al.: Development of carcinoma of the lung as reflected in exfoliated cells. Cancer, 33: 256–270, 1974.

Saccomanno, G.: Diagnostic Pulmonary Cytology, American Society of Clinical Pathologists, Chicago, 1978.

Sachs, H., Bahnsen, J. and Stegner, H.-E.: Scanning-mikroscopisch-cytometrische Untersuchungen und Dysplasien des Collum uteri. Arch. Gynäk., 212: 401–412, 1972.

Sachs, H., Stegner, H.-E. and Bahnsen, J.: Cytophotometrische Untersuchungen an Epitheldysplasien des Collum uteri. Arch. Gynäk., 212: 97–129, 1972.

Sachs, H. and Schäfer, E.: Feulgen DNS-Cytophotometrie an Zellabstrichen der Cervix uteri. Arch. Gynäk., 215: 171–186, 1973.

Saffiotti, U., Montesano, R., Sellakumar, A.R. and Borg, S.A.: Experimental cancer of the lung. Inhibition by vitamin A of the induction of tracheobronchial squamous metaplasia and squamous cell tumors. Cancer, 20: 857–864, 1967.

Saffiotti, U.: Role of Vitamins in Carcinogenesis. Amer. J. Clin. Nutri., 22(8) 1088, 1969.

Sandritter, W., Carl, M. and Ritter, W.: Cytophotometric Measurements of the DNA Content of Human Malignant Tumors by Means of the Feulgen Reaction. Acta Cytol., 10(1): 26–30, 1966.

Sato, H., Akaogi, E., Saito, Y. et al.: Transbronchial needle aspiration for lung cancer patients, especially for the cases in which cancer cells were negative in the specimens taken by the brushing method. J. Jap. Soc. Clin. Cytol., 16: 182–187, 1977. (in Japanese with English abstract)

Sawada, K., Akamine, Y., Miura, S. et al.: Aspiration biopsy smear of subcarinal lymphnode under bronchoscopy in bronchogenic carcinoma. Lung Cancer, 11: 3–9, 1971. (in Japanese with English abstract)

Sawada, K., Fukuma, S., Seki, Y. et al.: Giant cell carcinoma of the lung: Clinical and pathological correlation. Lung Cancer, 21: 395–403, 1981. (in Japanese with English abstract)

Schreiber, H., Saccomanno, G., Martin, D.H. and Brennan, L.: Sequential cytological changes during development of respiratory tract tumors induced in hamsters by benzo(a)pyrene ferric oxide. Cancer Res., 34: 689–698, 1974.

Shibata, H.: Annual Report of the Cancer Research, Ministry of Health and Welfare, 1982.

Sinner, W.N.: Transthoracic needle biopsy of small peripheral malignant lung lesions. Invest. Radiol., 8: 305–314, 1973.

Sinner, W.N.: Complications of percutaneous transthoracic needle aspiration biopsy. Acta. Radiol. (Diagnosis), 17: 813–828, 1976.

Sniffen, R.C., Soutter, L. and Robbins, L.L.: Muco-epidermoid tumors of the bronchus arising from surface epithelium. Amer. J. Pathol., 34: 671–683, 1958.

Söderström, N.: Fine Needle Aspiration Biopsy. Almqvist & Wiksell, Stockholm, 1966.

Spencer, H.: Pathology of the Lung, 3rd ed., Vol. 2, Pergamon Press, Oxford, 1977.

Stackhouse, E.M., Harrison, E.G. and Ellis, F.H.: Primary mixed malignancies of lung: Carcinosarcoma and blastoma. J. Thorac. Cardiovasc. Surg., 57: 385–399, 1969.

Stenbäck, F. and Sellakumar, A.: Squamous metaplasia and respiratory tumor induced by intratracheal instillation of 7, 12-dimethyl-(a)-anthracene in Syrian golden hamsters. Eur. J. Cancer, 10: 483–486, 1974.

Takahashi, M.: Respiratory tract. In: Color Atlas of Cancer Cytology, 2nd ed., Igaku-Shoin, Tokyo and New York, 1981. pp. 267–334.

Takemoto, T., Kawai, K., Ida, K. et al.: Techniques and Applications of Endoscopic Dyeing Method. Igaku-Tosho-Shuppan, Tokyo, 1976. (in Japanese)

Tipton, D.L. and Crocker, T.: Duration of Brochial Squamous Metaplasia Produced in Dogs by Cigarette Smoke Condensate. J. Nat. Cancer Inst., 33(3): 487–495, 1964.

Törzsök, L.: Die transbronchiale Punktion. Praxia Pneumol., 29: 162–165, 1975.

Tsuboi, E.: Atlas of Transbronchial Biopsy, Early Diagnosis of Peripheral Pulmonary Carcinomas, Igaku-Shoin Ltd., Tokyo, 1970.

Versteegh, R.M. and Swierenga, J.: Bronchoscopic evaluation of the operability of pulmonary carcinoma. Acta Oto-Laryngol., 56: 603–611, 1963.

Wagner, D., Richart, R.M. and Terner, J.Y.: Deoxyribonucleic Acid Content of Presumed Precursors of Endometrial Carcinoma. Cancer, 29: 2067–2077, 1967.

Westcott, J.L.: Air embolism complicating percutaneous needle biopsy of the lung. Chest, 63: 108–110, 1973.

W. H. O.: Biological effects of asbestos: Report of the Advisory Committee on Asbestos Cancers to the Director of the International Agency for Research on Cancer. Ann. Occup. Hyg., 16: 9–17, 1973.

W. H. O.: Histological Typing of Lung Tumours, International Histological Classification of Tumours, No. 1, 2nd ed., World Health Organization, Geneva, 1981.

Wolinsky, H. and Lishner, M.W.: Needle track implantation of tumor after percutaneous lung biopsy. Ann. Intern. Med., 71: 359–362, 1969.

Woolf, C.R.: Applications of aspiration lung biopsy with a review of the literature, Dis. Chest, 25: 286–301, 1954.

Woolner, L.B.: Pulmonary Cytology, Teaching Slide Sets in Cytology, Vol. 15, Tutorials of Cytology, Chicago, 1973.

Yoshida, M.: Endoscopic toluidine blue-iodine double staining method for an aid of detection and diagnosis of eroding lesion of the esophagus. Gastroenterological Endoscopy, 23: 1691–1703, 1981. (in Japanese with English abstract)

Zetterberg, A. and Esposti, P-L.: Cytophotometric DNA-Analysis of Aspirated Cells from Prostatic Carcinoma. Acta Cytol., 20(1): 46–57, 1976.

INDEX